THE 10 MINUTE MIRACLE

THE
1O MINUTE MIRACLE

The Quick Fix Survival
Guide for Mind & Body

Gloria Rawson
&
David Callinan

Thorsons
An Imprint of HarperCollins*Publishers*

Thorsons
An Imprint of HarperCollinsPublishers
77–85 Fulham Palace Road
Hammersmith, London W6 8JB

Published by Thorsons 1998
1 3 5 7 9 10 8 6 4 2

A catalogue record for this book
is available from the British Library

ISBN 0 7225 3658 5

Printed and bound in Great Britain by
Woolnough Bookbinding Ltd, Irthlingborough, Northants

CONTENTS

PREFACE

WHY 10 MINUTES, WHY A MIRACLE?

WHOEVER WE ARE, WHATEVER OUR CIRCUMstances, we have all lived through moments of what might be called 20th-century syndrome. Some of us are better able to deal with it than others, by facing problems square on, with grim determination. In fact stress and crises in our lives can often be a driving force, enabling us to win through a difficult or painful situation. It's only when stress builds up in our lives and we don't, won't or simply can't alter our way of thinking that it can cause damage. The tension starts to build up in our bodies, negative thoughts creep in, we start to feel below par, we get a headache, go off our food, feel out of sorts. This is the spiralling-down effect of modern life.

What we need to help us through our day-to-day challenges is a guide to self-healing which incorporates real knowledge within a fast-track approach. That's how the '10 Minute Miracle' was born. We decided to write this book, not for yogis, enlightened beings, saints or superstars, but for ordinary, everyday, rushed-off-their feet people who really are searching for ways to take control of their lives and their health. People like us and, maybe, like you.

How the '10 Minute Miracle' Works

The '10 Minute Miracle' is a self-help technique which shows you how to practise simple holistic survival therapies, both in isolation and as part of comprehensive routines.

Each section of the book takes you through the therapies themselves – affirmations, meditation, reflexology, chi kung, crystal power and so on – with background information (All About ...), practical guidance (Using the therapy to enhance your life), and the 10 minute miracle techniques themselves.

By spending just 10 minutes at a time practising these 10 minute routines, you can make a huge difference to your own health, your confidence, your ability to think positively (and not negatively) and your overall well-being.

Start to prepare yourself to change your life. This is the real miracle. When you can do this – when you can take charge of your own health and well-being – then you are on the way to a revelation.

Take it slowly. Learn each technique if you can. If you find some simply impossible to do, then don't worry. There is enough in this book to change everyone's life. When you feel confident you can practise the basics of each technique, start putting the 10 minute miracle combinations into practice. This is the first step in holistic programming, and it takes just 10 minutes. The healing power within you is already there. It's yours. Why not find it and use it?

AFFIRMATIONS

ALL ABOUT AFFIRMATIONS

LEARNING HOW TO MAKE AN AFFIRMATION IS like turning a key that opens the door. It is our chance to change something fundamental about our lives for the better – and for ever. But before we can make some changes in our lives, we need to look into how we see ourselves and how others see us.

Have there ever been moments when you've been tempted to think that life is treating you unfairly? Well, we've probably all experienced that feeling at one time or another in our lives.

One of the reasons that we so often fail to achieve our goals is that somehow we 'block' our ability to do so.

Something deep down within our own life condition is working in a negative response to outside forces, and although we may put in exhausting amounts of energy to achieve something, we don't quite make it. The result is often a crushing blow to our ego and to our hopes and dreams for a better life. When we keep getting knocked in this way, we start to give up on our goals, dreams and aspirations. This is a shame, because we all have great potential within us.

The Power to Change

We each have the power to change things and improve our lives beyond measure. We can begin from this moment in time. This power inside us is the very core of our own existence on this planet. We just need to learn how to honour and respect ourselves, our relationships and our environment (which is totally connected to us and which will respond to us if we ask). Once we know how, we can use our knowledge to its full potential, giving ourselves maximum exposure to the opportunities and openings that are out there for us.

A change from within creates a change from without.

Good Vibrations

Affirmations go to the very depths of our lives and change our way of thinking, so that we can unlock unlimited potential from within. By digging out all the negativity, we then allow in this pure creative vibration – called an affirmation.

USING AFFIRMATIONS TO ENHANCE YOUR LIFE

Make a List

You need to make up a list of the affirmations that are going to help you change your life. The first step is to take a pen and paper, sit quietly and write down all the things you are currently worried about, the issues that can keep you awake at night. Then create a list of the things that you have always wanted for yourself. This might contain your material assets, and your emotional needs. Don't be afraid to put down all your dreams. At first you might laugh at what you are writing down, but some things on your list will make you reflect a little on what it is you haven't been able to achieve or do, due to unforeseen obstacles that came in the way, or some other reason.

When compiling your list, you may become aware that the reason you haven't achieved some of your goals is a restrictive element (such as you never had enough money, encouragement, lacked confidence, no parental backing, partner didn't want you to). It is helpful if you list these reasons over on the right-hand side of the page.

Just by making this list you will start to analyse your own life, how you see yourself and what you want for the future.

Please put this book down now and make your list, before reading further, as this is the first step towards preparing yourself for your own very individual affirmations, which will enable you to change your life in every aspect, for ever.

The Power to Forgive

I forgive everyone, including myself.

Think of all the incidents throughout your early life, linked to teachers, relatives, parents, friends, people in authority, who at one time or another sent out the wrong signals. At the time you were trusting and heeded their actions, comments or criticisms. Then, having grown up and gone out into the world, you began to have your own experiences and could draw on them to form your own opinions, and then came to realize that you may have been misinformed in some ways, in your formative years. Some of these realizations are painful, especially, for example, if they involve your own family. But you need to try to see why your parents or carers may have taught you these things, and how you need no longer be bound by outdated or inappropriate thought patterns.

I love and accept myself exactly as I am.

It also helps to remember that everyone on this Earth has been a beautiful baby, a small innocent child. By using an affirmation where you FORGIVE YOURSELF, YOUR FAMILY, NO MATTER WHAT HAS HAPPENED IN THE

PAST, you can release negativity from deep within and set yourself free. You are then empowered.

How to Make an Affirmation

WORK WITH YOUR AFFIRMATIONS FIRST THING IN THE MORNING AND AGAIN IN THE EVENING.

You will need a small notebook to log your reactions to your affirmations. By logging your responses, you will be able to see not only a change in the way you think about yourself, but, in time, the way you think about other people. Soon, your recorded comments will start to show a more positive acknowledgement of the affirmation. Remember to date your comments.

Develop your own affirmations to suit your own needs. An affirmation is always expressed in the PRESENT TENSE. It must be written down and performed to yourself in front of the mirror each morning and evening, saying each affirmation three times, for at least 40 days. If you miss a day, you go back to day one in counting how many days you have completed. By the end of an unbroken run of 40 days, your outlook will have changed beyond recognition and you will then be able to drop some of the initial affirmations made. You can always re-introduce them at a later date, if you feel you still need to do a little more work on that particular area of your life. But after your 40 days you can confidently drop some of your original affirmations and create some new ones to help you with the new set of circumstances happening to you.

The Power of Your Voice

By voicing an affirmation three times, saying it to yourself not just once but three times, you begin the process of healing. You need to hear these positive words entering into your psyche. The sound of your voice is all important – you can't just think it.

As you begin to say your affirmations each day you will begin to realize just how empowering they are. You will be amazed at the speed in which your life will start to open up and change.

SAMPLE AFFIRMATIONS

Affirmation	*Notes on Reaction*
I am willing to change	I don't need to change
I love myself as I am	I hate myself as I am
I love … exactly as he/she is	He/she is the one who needs to change
I live in harmony with those I love	No I don't, we argue a lot
All in my world is well	It couldn't be worse right now
I am flexible and respond to new ideas	People don't seem to listen to me
There is plenty for everyone on this planet, including me	I'm so hard up these days
I move into an exciting new phase in my life	I am frightened of change

Here are some ideas on what you may want to affirm for:

- ★ A MORE POSITIVE OUTLOOK ON LIFE IN GENERAL
- ★ A CHANGE IN YOUR WORKING/LIVING ENVIRONMENT
- ★ A CHANGE IN YOUR RELATIONSHIPS
- ★ MORE SELF-ESTEEM, SELF-RESPECT, SELF-WORTH
- ★ MORE FRIENDS
- ★ MORE MONEY
- ★ MORE JOB OPPORTUNITIES.

Try to think of about a dozen or so affirmations on the self-changing theme and stick to them (remember, 40 days). After 40 days the changes in your life should be noticeable and you will already be thinking about other affirmations to add to your list. It is always OK to add new affirmations to an existing list (just add the date you put them on the list; then you will know when you have been affirming them for 40 days).

Your affirmations can address any area of your life you wish: your job/career, relationships, money-making, your dreams and desires. Once you have begun your self-work, with affirmations and the other techniques in this book to create a 10 minute miracle workout each day, your life will begin to unfold in the most interesting way.

I acknowledge the obstacles in my life are an opportunity to change from within.

I accept these challenges and overcome them one by one, expediently and with ease.

If it's right for your life and you affirm for it in the way described here, then you WILL start to realize all you want in your life.

A 10 MINUTE MIRACLE

★ Make sure you are quite alone (because you do not want to be hampered by self-consciousness or discomfort in any way).

★ Use a mirror. Stand in front of it and look directly into your own eyes.

★ Repeat your chosen affirmation THREE TIMES, saying the affirmation to yourself as you look in the mirror.

You may feel you want to burst into tears, or you may be angry (especially if you just don't believe what you're affirming). Don't allow a reaction like this to stop you from carrying on – it does get easier each time you do it.

Try the following affirmations, or devise your own to suit your situation. For this first experience of affirmations, use the entire 10 minutes just to reinforce your newfound habit. After a time, you can incorporate affirmations into some of the other 10 minute miracle routines as discussed later in this book.

I am balanced and at one with the universe.

I am focused and full of wonderful energy.

I feel love and compassion for everyone, especially (name of person).

Say the affirmations with real feeling three times, remembering to have that trusty notebook handy to jot down your reactions. You will find it illuminating later on to see how your reactions have changed. It may take time. The suggested period, as mentioned, is 40 days. This allows the affirmation to penetrate your subconscious and enable changes to occur naturally. Don't forget to write down your affirmations in advance under daily headings. Affirmations are the key to everything in your life changing. You maximise these changes by selecting a daily 10 minute miracle.

2

AROMATHERAPY

I am open to the healing potential of essential oils.

ALL ABOUT AROMATHERAPY

What Are 'Essential' Oils?

THEY ARE OFTEN CALLED THE LIFE-FORCE, or life 'blood' of a plant. These essences are extracted from the bark, leaf, berry, fruit or flower of a tree, bush or plant, usually by distillation or cold pressing.

Choosing an Essential Oil

There are over 130 different essential oils. This chapter describes just a few of the most commonly used and some of their properties.

ALL ESSENTIAL OILS HAVE THE CAPACITY WITHIN THEM TO HELP ENHANCE YOUR LIFE AT ALL TIMES. ALL ESSENTIAL OILS HELP BOOST YOUR IMMUNE SYSTEM. ALL HELP BALANCE YOU EMOTIONALLY, MENTALLY AND PHYSICALLY.

Where You Can Find Essential Oils

You can buy essential oils in most good high street chemists, gift and speciality shops or by mail order from health and lifestyle magazines.

Usually the oils are sold in 5- or 10-ml bottles, and should be kept in a cool dark place, to ensure that the vitality of the oil is not lost. Dark-coloured bottles are used to assist in this process. The oils are volatile and will need to be blended into a 'carrier' oil (a vegetable-based oil) before they are used on the body.

Safety Tips

★ Avoid sunbathing after you have had an aromatherapy session. Also avoid the use of a sun bed. Essential oils may cause burning if the skin is exposed to direct sunlight after treatment.

★ Always treat the oils with respect. The small amounts indicated are all you need. It is unnecessary to use more than the required amount. Overdosing can be harmful, it can cause slight burning of the skin, so don't be tempted to use more than 3 drops per 5 ml carrier oil (or 3%).

★ Pregnant women should not use oils during the first four months of pregnancy. After four months, the two oils most commonly used during pregnancy are Mandarin and Lavender – but in VERY LOW PERCENTAGES – usually 1 drop of essential oil to 5 ml of carrier oil (1%) or even 1 drop of essential oil to 10 ml of carrier oil (.5%).

★ If you are put off by the smell of a blend, add a little Lavender to it. Often a blend will smell better once carrier oil is added to it – otherwise, start again.

If in doubt about the use of oils and if you suffer from a particular ailment or condition, consult a qualified aromatherapist.

DO NOT allow the top of the bottle to come into contact with the skin. Always tip the bottle and let the droplet fall onto the palm of the hand, in a bowl, saucer, or onto a tissue.

USING AROMATHERAPY TO ENHANCE YOUR LIFE

So you've bought a selection of oils and taken them home – what now?

A 10 MINUTE MIRACLE

In the Bath

I am absorbed totally in warmth and luxury.

When choosing a blend for your bath, first you have to ask yourself – HOW DO I FEEL? Am I tired, achy, worried about something? Essential oils are very good for alleviating aches, and are comforting. Equally they can be invigorating and can actually help you to concentrate; they can be a wonderfully refreshing way to start the day as well. It's fun to make up your own blends, but of course you run the risk of ending up with something that isn't always the best of smells and the different oils may then seem to be struggling for their own identity, rather than complementing one another.

Lavender is a good all-round oil and is very useful in bringing the blend together. Remember when blending, it is sometimes better to let one oil dominate, so use more drops of that oil. But consider too that just 1 drop of an oil can change a blend dramatically, so it is best to start off with, say, two different oils together, then three and so on. Three oils are usually a good basis for a pleasing bath blend.

Here are a few blends that will start you off, added to 1 dessert spoon of milk or 1 teaspoon of vodka, or 1 teaspoon of carrier oil:

BATH BLENDS TO START THE DAY
★ 2 drops Geranium, 2 Juniper, 1 Lemon
★ 2 drops Rosemary, 1 Lemon, 2 Grapefruit
★ 2 drops Grapefruit, 1 Lemon, 1 Geranium

TO SOOTHE ACHING MUSCLES
★ 2 drops Chamomile, 2 Lavender, 1 Clary Sage
★ 2 drops Chamomile, 2 Bergamot, 1 Lavender
★ 2 drops Chamomile, 2 Bergamot, 1 Marjoram

ROMANTIC BATH BLENDS FOR YOU AND YOUR PARTNER
★ 2 drops Jasmine, 2 Sandalwood, 1 Clary Sage
★ 2 drops Rose, 2 Sandalwood, 1 Patchouli
★ 2 drops Jasmine, 2 Ylang Ylang, 1 Bergamot

★ 3 drops Patchouli, 3 Frankincense

★ 2 drops Marjoram, 2 Lavender. Also can be used for massage: 2 drops Marjoram, 1 drop Lavender per 5 ml carrier oil. Marjoram assists in dilating blood vessels and helps to speed up healing in an injured limb.

In the Shower

Although there's often nothing to beat having a soothing bath using essential oils, you can use them when taking a shower very quickly and easily. First dampen a clean flannel with warm water. Use one oil and place 3 drops onto the flannel, then fold over. Rub your body with the flannel and then take your shower in the usual way, using your favourite soap or shower gel. The essential oil will work its way through your skin as the heat from the shower water cascades over you.

Jacuzzi

If you have a jacuzzi, essential oils can be used and are far superior to the chemical compounds normally used in the recycled water of a public jacuzzi. Bear in mind also that the antiseptic quality of all essential oils will protect you, so doesn't it make good sense to use them, especially if you like to share the experience with someone, or a group of people?

Sauna

The best oils for use in the sauna are Lemon, Pine, Lime or Rosemary. Reason – because these oils help eliminate toxins from the body, via the skin. The oils should be added with the water which is thrown on the coals, or whatever method of heating the sauna.

A 10 MINUTE MIRACLE

Relieving Colds, Catarrh, Sinusitis

I quickly respond to the healing qualities of nature's medicines.

This 10 minute routine may resemble old-fashioned remedies for the above ailments. Nevertheless, when combined with essential oils, this method never fails to bring relief.

PREPARATION

Take a large Pyrex or glazed ceramic bowl (not plastic as the essential oil may damage it). Pour very hot water into the bowl and drop approximately 3–4 drops of a chosen oil or blend of oils into the water. The oils will float on top of the water. Now, take a towel and cover your head, leaning over the bowl and inhale deeply. Come up for air occasionally and then repeat several times. The feeling is not unlike that of a facial sauna. This technique is good for your skin too.

A little word of warning here: If you have broken veins on your face, please be careful and don't do this treatment for too long. Equally you can try to protect the broken veins with a little Vaseline over them before you start to inhale.

Here are some suggested blends you can use as remedies:

★ Bad cold – 2 drops Eucalyptus, 1 Peppermint, 1 Tea tree
★ Catarrh, sinus congestion – 2 drops Eucalyptus, 1 Peppermint, 1 Pine
★ Coughs – 2 drops Hyssop, 1 Frankincense, 1 Marjoram

Sore Throat

This method is a little different. Lay a flannel in hot water, not as hot as the bowl method, into which you have put 2 drops of Hyssop, 1 drop of Lavender and 1 drop of Clary Sage. Because essential oils are not water-soluble, they will float on top of the water and vapourize into the flannel, Just wrap the flannel around your throat and leave till it cools. Repeat several times. This is remarkably warming and comforting.

Healing Other Minor Ailments, Cuts and Bruises

If you carry a bottle of Lavender oil with you, you can treat cuts and bruises in an emergency. It can act as a useful form of smelling salts, if you, or someone else has had an accident or is in shock.

★ For wounds, sores and cuts – 1 drop Lavender and 1 Neroli in a carrier oil: apply to the area once it has been cleaned thoroughly

★ Migraine, PMS – 1 drop Peppermint on a tissue. Alternatively, massage your temples lightly with a little Lavender (one drop) rubbed on the fingers of both hands. This helps to alleviate tension.

★ Bruising – 1 drop Lavender, 1 Geranium, 1 Rosemary, all diluted in 5 ml carrier oil, applied directly to the bruise. Treat daily.

Candle Burners

These are ceramic pots with a space at the base to place a small tee light or candle designed for this purpose (in an aluminium pocket). Essential oil molecules are released into the air by heat, engulfing smells and odours and destroying them, as well as airborne germs. Can be used at home and in your office or workplace.

Electric burners are an alternative to ceramic ones. You simply plug them in and they can be left on for long periods. This type of burner maintains an even level of heat.

A 10 MINUTE MIRACLE

I am in harmony with those I love and work with.

Here are some ideas for using oils in a burner for everyday situations.

* ★ To help you calm down after an argument or shock – Melissa and Ylang Ylang
* ★ Cleansing the air you breathe – Lavender, Geranium and Bergamot

★ Enhancing your work environment, for colleagues as well as yourself – Lavender, Juniper and Bergamot
★ Harmonizing the 'atmosphere' after an argument or disagreement – Lavender and Bergamot
★ To help pep up a flagging relationship with a partner – Sandalwood and Ylang Ylang
★ Eradicating bad odours (such as cooking smells) – Lavender, Geranium and Bergamot (or for particularly stubborn or obnoxious odours, burn Lemon and Lime together)
★ Killing airborne germs and purifying the air – Lavender and Tea tree
★ To help protect you from illness, if someone close to you is not well – Lavender and Tea tree
★ Lifting your mood if you are feeling down – Select two of the following: Bergamot, Neroli, Jasmine, Rose, Sandalwood, Ylang Ylang or Clary-Sage
★ To make social events go with a swing – Orange and Bay oils are warming; Lavender and Bergamot are relaxing and uplifting. Try your own combinations for fun – you never know what the results might be.

★ To combat hay fever – any of the following: Chamomile, Lavender, Lemon, Peppermint, Rosemary. Also, 1 drop Chamomile on a tissue and kept with you will help.

★ To ease anxiety – Bergamot, Jasmine, Lavender, Ylang Ylang or Rosewood (singly or pick two). Also good in self-massage. It also helps to put a few drops on a tissue which you will not use other than for inhaling. Keep it near to you and every few minutes take a deep breath in as you hold the tissue to your nose.

★ General illness – Tea tree is a great immune booster, used in a burner, the bath, on a tissue or inhaled.

For those times when you haven't access to a burner:

★ Keeping the car fresh – a few drops of Lemon oil on a cotton ball. Put the wad somewhere in your car and you will be amazed at how alert and refreshed you feel while driving.

★ Alertness when driving, by night or when tired – a few drops of Peppermint, Lemon and Rosemary on a cotton bud before you set out on your journey. If you begin to feel tired and start nodding off at the wheel, just inhale the fragrances and you will feel rejuvenated. Turn the car heater off and open a window slightly too.

★ Travelling generally – put a drop of Lavender oil on a tissue and take it with you when travelling. It helps keep you calm in rush hours, may prevent the onset of road rage and help you cope with packed buses, trains held up by signals, road works and traffic jams.

AROMATHERAPY MASSAGE: A 10 MINUTE MIRACLE

The healing properties of essential oils protect me and the environment I live and work in at all times.

Preparation

You can massage most of your body easily in 10 minutes, sitting on a towel on the floor. Please make sure that you are comfortable. If necessary, place an eiderdown or duvet on the floor, covered with some towels or a sheet.

Make sure the room is warm and have to hand some tissues in case of spillage, and a saucer to pour some oil out if you don't wish to decant straight into your hand.

Put on some soothing music, if you like (*see Chapter 10*). Now you're ready.

★ Take up some ready-blended essential oil in a good carrier oil (remember, no more than 3 drops per 5-ml of carrier oil) and cover the palm of one hand.

★ Use a stroking movement initially, travelling along the outside of one arm, over the shoulder and along the neckline, to the base of the scalp. Then, glide down and over the front of your shoulder and down the inside of the upper arm and then down to the palm of the hand. Repeat this twice more, on the third time gently squeezing and releasing the muscles as you go.

★ Repeat on the other arm, and then each leg, using long sweeping movements down the front of the leg and up the back, gently squeezing and releasing the calf and thigh muscles en route. Be gentle over the knee area, at the front and back.

★ Include your feet in the massage, going in between the toes and oiling the base of the foot as well.

★ For women, massage the breast area, using light, gentle circular movements – holding the breasts for a few moments. For men, massage the chest area by following the rib cage downwards with fingertip movements and then a circular action, using the palms of both hands over the whole area two or three times.

★ For the solar plexus and abdomen, use a circular movement with the palms in contact in a clockwise direction several times. This can be a very sensitive area for some, especially those who are highly strung or nervy. It is important to go fairly slowly over the whole area, making sure the oil is quite warm. The ancient art of Chi Kung (*see page 56*) recommends massage in this area should be clockwise for women and anti-clockwise for men.

★ Stand up and massage your buttocks, going as far up your back as you can, a few times. This will incorporate the area of the kidneys.

★ Place one oiled palm over the opposite shoulder and massage down the blade as far as you can. Repeat with the other palm on the other shoulder.

★ Finally, use a few small circular movements with the fingers and thumbs in the hairline and scalp. This is deeply relaxing. The oil is very beneficial to your hair and scalp – if you can, leave the oil on overnight (wrapping your head in a towel) and wash it out in the morning.

Take your time over this. If you cram in more strokes, you will feel exhausted. It is far better to go slowly and do a few strokes, allowing the essential oils to soak in.

Now you've learned how simple it is to use essential oils in a variety of ways to make your life healthier and more fulfilling. Do allow yourself to experiment.

3

VISUALIZATION

ALL ABOUT VISUALIZATION

YOUR IMAGINATION, COUPLED WITH FOCUSED desire and intention, is one of the most powerful tools you possess. The light that comes from the sun is diffuse, touching everything. When focused to the point of a laser, it can cut through steel. What we will now learn is how to spend 10 minutes or even less, turning our imagination into a laser.

Because you are going to learn and practise how to focus your creative energy, you will be able to use the technique in many ways – particularly when it comes to those things you truly desire, the life situation which you know will make you happy and fulfilled. This need not be money or fame – in most cases true contentment and fulfilment come from much deeper and more profound desires than these.

USING VISUALIZATION TO ENHANCE YOUR LIFE

The process of visualization enables you to create a clear image or feeling in your mind and to give that image energy and reality. The key is to repeat the process over and over again. It works for both short-term and long-term life situations. If you are about to go into an important job interview, or make an important proposal, or decide to make that approach to someone you like, then you can improve the situation and bring positive energy to bear by visualizing the situation and how you would like to see it developing.

Your goal may be on the physical level – you may be ill, run down, anxious or depressed. It can be on an emotional level – you've had an argument with someone you work with or love, or you are trying to find a way to tell someone something painful. It might be mental – you have to take a difficult exam or test, or you may have to face a complicated business situation. Or it could even be spiritual – your desire to grow spiritually and psychically, to understand your own cosmic being and your relationship with existence and beyond.

Here are some examples which might relate to your own personal experience, and which can be helped with creative visualization:

★ You are having a problem with someone you care about
★ The boss (or a work colleague) is an absolute tyrant
★ You suffer from headaches or other stress-related conditions
★ You want to restore balance, harmony, calm and confidence within yourself
★ You want to feel more connected to your environment
★ You want to enhance your general health and well-being

Visualization Techniques – The Basics

Start with an affirmation such as:

I visualize the situation I desire.

For each of the visualizations that follow, find a quiet place and get comfortable. Try to sit with a straight back, against a wall or in a chair or on the floor. Let your hands rest easily on your lap, close your eyes and listen to your breathing. Don't try to stop thoughts as they come.

Know what you want to happen, or what you want to achieve. When you are in a deeply relaxed state of mind, begin to see the situation as though it is actually happening now. You might like to tape-record yourself (or a friend) reading the '10 Minute Miracle' techniques in this chapter, to play back while you are first trying out the visualizations.

As you get more proficient, you can begin to use the techniques in the midst of a crowd, sitting on a bus or a train or waiting on a platform, or in almost any situation.

10 MINUTE MIRACLES

Starting Your Day

Let a golden ball of light descend on you from above. Just let the light bathe you in its golden warmth. Allow the light to pass down your body and let yourself relax. Breathe slowly and deeply. If it helps, count down to one from 20 or 10. Now, just picture the place you are in, wherever it is. See it in your mind's eye. See yourself sitting in this room or place, and really look at the room in your mind. Examine every corner of the room, the windows and doors. If you can't hold a picture in your mind, just think about the room. The pictures will come of their own accord. Tell yourself how happy you now are to be here – whatever has happened in the past. Affirm to yourself that you have been truly happy here. You can remember some nice things that have happened in the room, recall pleasant or really pleasurable experiences.

Now you are on the move. The walls of the room are transparent and, whatever the weather outside, you are travelling, up and away, over rooftops and houses, over parks and gardens, swooping down along motorways and familiar places. You are in control and you are safe, in your own world. When you feel you want to return, just come slowly back to home, say goodbye to your happy room and vow you will return again soon for another magic carpet ride.

Visualization and Health

Imagine any tension you feel as a sprung coil unwinding and leaving you. Feel a deep relaxation taking its place. When you are relaxed, imagine you are standing outside a wondrous building. It can be large or small, on a tropical island or on a distant planet – whatever enters your mind, let it be. Don't question or apply logic or reason. You know this building is your own personal health clinic. Only you can enter, and inside you know you will find the key to health and well-being. If you suffer from a complaint, illness or disease in which your body is out of tune with the environment – or out of balance in any way, tell yourself that the answers lie inside this building.

Enter the building and walk into a beautiful environment. Forget all preconceptions. The room is filled with light of different colours. Walk towards the colour which attracts you. Within this colour you find a white bed. Lie on the bed and welcome your own personal physician. You know that this person has your best interests at heart and wondrous skills. The physician places hands upon you and asks you what help you need. You recount exactly how you feel. This person's fingers trace over your body but you feel the effects in your soul. You feel wonderful. This is your visualized psychic physician who knows you intimately and who can bring you true healing power. A ball of light will surround the area which needs attention.

You are in wonderful hands and are in perfect health, bursting with vitality. When you feel it is time to go, thank your physician and leave in peace, feeling wonderful and knowing you can return whenever you wish.

Coping with Stress

Imagine yourself stepping out from your own body – turning around and facing yourself, so you are looking at your own image. It is important to learn to do this before you go on to the next step. Hold this image of yourself in your mind. Take your time.

Imagine a golden white flow of pure energy entering this image of yourself through the temples. This golden white energy flows into and fills every part of the body before you. Witness the fact that you are standing in front of yourself and you are watching yourself fill up with golden white light.

As the golden white light fills every single corner of your image, it is also cleansing it and restoring it to health. Now you notice that the golden white light flows out through the feet of your image – so now you have this constant flow of energy ... entering through your temples, filling up your whole body and then leaving through your feet.

Imagine too that the energy that leaves through your feet becomes cleansed again as it takes away all the impurities and imbalances from your body and gets recycled and re-absorbed as pure golden white energy again ... like a cycle of never-ending energy, your image takes in this energy, which cleanses your body, taking with it any debris out through the soles of your feet, to then become cleansed and return as pure white energy once more ... entering your temples and filling your whole body image.

Keep this process of recycled pure white energy flowing through your body image for as long as you wish. When you feel you have done this for long enough, simply imagine the closing over of the temples and the feet, the energy then being CONTAINED in the body image. Now just imagine your image walking towards you, slowly coming forward and merging with you once more. Notice how good this feeling is and hold on to that wonderful feeling of pure energy and joy. Gradually stretch your arms and legs. Now open your eyes.

Imagine a golden ball of light literally rolling through you, slowly. The ball is going to penetrate every part of you like a magic magnet, right down into your very fibre. Here you will find your physical tension. Here you will discover the 'twisted' nerve endings. You may start to shake slightly as the ball permeates through your neck and shoulders. Let it collect the twisted, jangling shivers of nervous energy. Visualize the stress, and the reasons for the stress if you know them, getting stuck to the ball as it works through you, cleansing your system.

When the ball has reached your feet, let it roll away into nothingness. Then imagine a soft, warm wind or breeze invigorating and refreshing the whole of your body. Let it blow right through you, quite hard and strong. Let it blow away the tension that remains. Let it blow away and scatter all the anxieties that have led you to this situation.

When you feel the time is right, let the wind vanish across the horizon or across a blue ocean. Slowly come out of your deep relaxation. Take a few slow and deep breaths and open your eyes, then return to your waking condition.

Enhancing Personal Relationships

Picture the person or the relationship situation you are in. Hold a picture in your mind, or hold the thought in your mind which sums up for you the situation, as clearly as you can. (This clarity is important.) When you are deeply relaxed you will find you are better able to pinpoint your focus. Create a scenario for yourself in which you are in a positive situation with this person. Imagine a conversation you would like to have, and affirm in the present tense that this is actually happening. Don't wish it to happen; visualize it actually happening. Tell yourself in your visualized state that you are truly relating in a positive and meaningful way with the other person, or that he or she is paying you real attention. Visualize yourself being close to someone you love or want to love. Visualize and pour energy into a situation with someone with whom you may be having difficulty. Visualize all this as though it is actually happening.

Visualization and Your Deepest Desires

Imagine you are entering a large bubble. This is your own personal prosperity bubble. Now you can visualize actually having exactly what you want or being the kind of person or living in the kind of life situation you most desire. This is not a wish. You must pour all your power into the visualized state, which must be here and now. You have achieved it. This is what it feels like to be where you want to be.

You can imagine a world or universe inside your personal bubble, which is protecting your desires from the elemental forces outside. You cannot be touched. Here you can be, or have, whatever you most desire. Remember, you are not wishing, you are experiencing the reality of what you want most.

When the moment is right, and only you will know when that moment comes, release the bubble and let go of it. Watch it ascend into the cosmos with all your desires locked inside it. Now you can rest assured in the knowledge that you will attract from the universe that which you truly need to make you happy.

It is important to realize that it is by repeating these visualization sessions that you will begin to see results. Simply sitting and wishing for something will not make it magically take place. Visualization is actually a voyage of self-discovery. Tearing down preconceived ideas about yourself can lead you to find out what you truly want and desire, as opposed to what you thought you wanted. This is a powerful developmental tool to achieve wealth, status or a particular relationship.

4

MEDITATION

ALL ABOUT MEDITATION

IMAGINE PERFECT PEACE. IMAGINE LIVING FOR the moment – the only time you really have.

Meditation is best described as overcoming outer perceptions in favour of inner awareness. It starts with thinking, as does every action we ever take. This leads to reflection, and then to inspiration. Initial thought disappears, non-stop thought processes cease and this in turn leads to a greater feeling of happiness and eventually to an experience of oneness with the universe. Beyond this point lies the ultimate form of perception, where the distinction between the meditator and the experienced object disappears. With meditation you can explore the cosmos, experience tranquillity and peace, lower your heart rate, improve your health, combat stress and blend all this with other techniques in this book.

USING MEDITATION TO ENHANCE YOUR LIFE

I change my awareness and my world changes too!

The key to meditating is to 'let go'.

Find a quiet, comfortable place to practise. It is possible to meditate on a bus or in a taxi, but it will take experience to do so since distractions, noise, clamour, crowds and all manner of activities will jog your mind out of the correct groove.

The ideal position for meditating is to sit on the floor with your back straight and your legs crossed but comfortable. If this is not possible, sit with your back straight in a firm but comfortable chair with your hands on your thighs, palm upwards and your feet placed flat on the ground.

1O MINUTE MIRACLES

Practice Breathing Session

As you close your eyes, let your body relax. Focus on the shoulders and imagine a stream of golden light pouring slowly down from above over your head and shoulders, entering your body and refreshing and relaxing you as it works its way down to your feet. Just keep your mind focused on the light and let thoughts come and go – no matter what they are, don't try to stop thinking.

As the light descends, follow it with your mind, allowing your mind to become one with the light.

You will notice your breathing has already slowed and, even now, physical changes are taking place. Allow yourself to become aware of your breathing. Recognize that this is the very stuff of life, of your very existence. You are taking then giving back, taking then giving back. It has been said that the very process of breathing, if fully understood and fully experienced, could teach us more than all the philosophies of the world.

Simply breathe through your nose, filling the diaphragm, then push the air downwards gently and then allow it to rise along your spine, upwards towards the crown of your head and then down the front of your body and out. This is called Inner Sky Breathing and it should become a natural breathing routine.

As you focus on your breathing you will experience a great calm. Allow thoughts to freely enter your mind, don't fight them. Begin now to really feel your body. Feel the energy of your breath spreading throughout your body and watch as thoughts subside. A moment will come when you are perfectly aware and perfectly calm and where thought has vanished. You will find yourself suspended, so to speak, in a thought-free zone and yet you will be aware of yourself. You will be aware that you are not your thoughts.

Allow your energy to flow into the earth, rooting you deep inside the planet, and imagine a silver thread pushing its way up out of the Earth and up along your spine and out of the crown of your head. Let yourself become suspended from that silver thread.

You will now feel deeply relaxed. Your body may react. Sometimes you may shudder, sometimes there will be involuntary reactions, such as a silent scream as tension starts to unwind from your nervous system and release itself from you. Let it happen. Fight nothing. Let the thoughts come again but this time be aware that they are thoughts, pushing into your mind. You are a calm centre. Listen to your breathing. Be at one with your breath.

Gradually you will allow yourself to come out of this meditative state. It is at this point that you will realize just how 'far' you are away from everyday consciousness as thoughts, sounds, memories, deadlines and noise start to assail you. When you finally open your eyes, rest awhile, allowing the everyday world to gradually filter back. To come back too quickly can jar the senses.

First Steps into Meditating

Become aware of your breath and allow a deep breath in very slowly ... as long as you can inhale, then hold the breath for a count of three: 1-2-3 ... Now release the breath, evenly, expelling all the air from your lungs, breathing out for as long as you can, until every last drop of air has been released ... and hold for a count of three: 1-2-3 ... Breathe in again and repeat the sequence, this time allowing your breathing to go deep and take longer inhaling, and slowly this time holding the breath count 1-2-3, then slowly releasing the breath and holding for a count of three 1-2-3. Do this two or three times more. Your breathing will be taking on a wonderful slow, steady rhythm and each sequence of breathing in can now be done through your nose, holding the breath and then releasing it slowly through your mouth, each time making sure you are performing this slowly. Going on from here, you can also incorporate the following thought with each in and out-breath: On the in-breath, imagine positive energy flooding into your body, holding it for a count of 1-2-3 ... and on the out-breath, release all the negative thoughts and feelings you may have – at the same time turning this negative into positive energy, holding for a count of 1-2-3. Again, breathe in positive energy, hold 1-2-3 ... breathe out negative energy and restore it to positive, hold 1-2-3.

This is a beneficial way to quiet your mind and slow things down; it is also your first step into meditating.

Meditating with Colour

Start your meditation the same way as before with the in-breath, holding for a count of 1-2-3 ... and then breathing out, holding for a count of 1-2-3.

Imagine a beautiful flower in the softest of yellows, directly in front of you. On the in-breath feel yourself entering the yellow flower. On the out-breath, allow this experience to float through you. Again on the in-breath, feel yourself and the flower merging together in all this wonderful yellowness. Be aware of the heavenly scent of this flower, its freshness – and note too how soft its petals are against your skin. On the out-breath, feel the experience. Focus on this one thing only now, as you continue your breathing. You may begin to breathe less deeply as you hold this one thought of the yellowness. Stay in this moment for as long as you need to.

When you wish to come out of the meditation, begin to concentrate on your in-breath and on your out-breath, as you gradually come back into reality. Before opening your eyes, start to be aware of the room and where you are sitting. Now slowly open your eyes.

You may repeat this meditation with other colours. The idea of the flower is that it is a focal point initially, and as you and the flower envelope one another, your mind enters a different realm.

Meditating with a Mantra

A mantra is a sound which, of itself, has no meaning but which can help induce a meditative state (*see page 146, Sounds Amazing*). Ancients believed that mantras contained special vibratory and spiritual qualities.

The sound can vary, but mantras such as 'Om', 'Ah', 'Hum', 'Hrih' are ancient sounds which can be used singly or in sequence. You might also try using your own name. If you do, you will find that it eventually becomes mere sound, devoid of its everyday associations and meaning. This can help refresh your view of yourself, giving you a new perspective.

Focus on your breathing and allow your thoughts to flow freely through your mind. You will feel or sense the right moment to begin repeating the sound or mantra to yourself.

If you use 'Om', for instance, let the sound stretch and shorten, expand and diminish as it will. Don't force it to appear or disappear. As the mantra is repeated, thoughts may intervene. Allow them free access. You will become aware that you, the real you, is monitoring the thought processes of your mind as though you are dissociated from them. Let the mantra continue, rising and falling, swelling and diminishing. Then thoughts will intrude again. Try to watch as a thought first bubbles up, even if it is the thought that you are meditating. As you practise your meditation the moments of absence of thought gradually increase. You will be suspended in a void, but not an empty void, one which is full of all potential.

Come out of the mantra when you feel you want to, then spend a few moments in non-thought mode before slowly letting yourself become aware of the outside world.

A 10 MINUTE MIRACLE

Combining Affirmation, Meditation and Aromatherapy

This 10 minute session involves a short aromatherapy massage (just the arms, legs and feet) combined with a brief but powerful affirmation and five minutes of meditation.

PREPARATION

★ You can have a bath or shower if you have time.

★ Lavender and Geranium oils; in an oil burner

★ Aromatherapy massage blend: 2–3 drops Juniper, Lemon and, say, Geranium (no more than this) with 5 ml carrier oil (Almond/Grapeseed/Peach Kernel/Sunflower/Safflower) in a small bowl

★ Towel or duvet to sit on

In your little sanctum or personal space, burn some Lavender and Geranium. This will help you to focus on an aspect of your life which you may have been unwilling or unprepared to face. The fragrances will seep into you, healing, comforting, reassuring. Accept them wholeheartedly, let them feel part of your being.

Make sure the room is warm but not over hot.

As well as the fragrant oils perfuming your room or space, you may wish to play some relaxing music (*see page 143, Sounds to Listen To*).

Sit in a relaxed position in front of a mirror. This mirror is going to become your confidante and your friend. You will have given some thought to your affirmation. It will be in the present tense, as always, and it will propose that whatever you are wishing for or suffering from has already been fulfilled or cured.

Look into the mirror and look deeply into your own eyes. Make your affirmation. Even if in your heart you simply do not believe it, make sure that while you are looking into your eyes and making the affirmation that, at that moment, you wholeheartedly believe what you are saying.

As with every affirmation, note down your immediate and instinctive reaction. Your reaction, at the moment you jot it down, may reflect deep inner disbelief or cynicism. No matter, stay true to the technique. It works, it really does.

AROMATHERAPY

Start with your arms. Take a little of the blended oil and use stroking movements up the outside of one arm, over the shoulder and neck, then glide down inside your arm to your hand. Gently massage your hand. There are many pressure points here. Using your thumb, simply circle around the palm and up along each finger. Repeat this three times, squeezing your muscles and tendons very gently on the last pass. Then repeat for your other arm.

When you massage your legs, use the same long sweeping movements down the front of the leg and up the back. As you slide your hand along the back of your legs, apply gentle pressure to the calf muscles, squeezing and releasing. Do not apply too much pressure on your knees. It is better to massage gently with your fingertips around the kneecap.

Finally, massage the feet. This will not be the same pressure-point technique as used in reflexology or shiatsu but more of an overall massage, over each foot, massaging each toe separately and applying a gentle wringing movement along the instep. Don't forget the heels. You can lightly pinch the outer side of each heel. Go over each foot three times.

MEDITATION

Sit comfortably and breathe slowly and easily, feeling warm and relaxed. For the moment we will choose the mantric sound HREE-AAH.

Let your mind float free. Allow yourself to be consciously aware of your thoughts. Recognize them as such: 'What's the time?'; 'I hope the car will start.' You will be amazed by the sheer number and sheer blather of your thoughts and equally interested to realize that you, the real you, is in some way separate from them. When you feel this, think it. Start the mantra, allowing it to rise and fall, weaken or strengthen, elongate and reverberate or shorten and vanish. Don't force anything. A moment will come (and it may only be the briefest of moments) when your thoughts and the mantra will stop, but your conscious self will remain. You will feel still and centred and aware that you encompass the universe, the macrocosm and the microcosm. Then thoughts may begin again and interrupt the flow, so start up the mantra once more.

Five minutes will pass very quickly, although you may experience time differently in your newly heightened state. You will be creating feelings of great peace in these still moments. Be patient. This is not an immediate guaranteed path to instant enlightenment, although moments of oneness with the universe will come. The key is just do it, without expectation or stress. Impose nothing on yourself. Do not intellectualize or question. Just be.

5

CHI KUNG

ALL ABOUT CHI KUNG

*C*HI IS WHAT THE CHINESE CALL ENERGY, THE energy of the universe of which we are part. Chi Kung is closely related to Tai Chi Chu'an, a martial art. This chapter will concentrate on a number of very simple Tai Chi stretches and Chi Kung exercises.

Many claims for improved health, longevity, joint rehabilitation, stress relief, the strengthening of internal organs and increased vitality are made for Chi Kung, and not without basis in fact. Many medical practitioners, such as osteopaths and chiropractors, approve of Tai Chi and Chi Kung as being supremely beneficial on the physical level.

On the question of warnings, some people find that practising Chi Kung can sometimes make them light-headed, a bit dizzy or even 'spaced out'. If this happens at any time then stop immediately, sit down and relax, or better still, lie down and practise deep relaxation.

The First Thing to Know – How to Stand

The first position is to stand with your feet in line with your hips, knees slightly bent. Relax your shoulders and distribute your weight evenly. Your arms should hang loose, elbows slightly bent and with a slight space under your armpits, so that your arms are held slightly out from the body. Keep the spine straight and the neck and head held up gently but firmly.

Imagine your feet are growing roots right down into the Earth. Then imagine a silver thread shooting up from the depths of the Earth, right up along your spine, out the top of your head and then on into the universe. The string lifts you slightly so that your head feels suspended from it – but comfortably.

Place your tongue on the roof of your mouth, just behind your teeth, and breathe through your nose, focusing on the base of the abdomen, beneath the solar plexus – what the Chinese call the *Tan Tien*. This is a point about one and a half inches below the navel. Let your breath fill this area first, then move up to your chest. The *Tan Tien* is the body's centre of gravity and a storehouse of Chi energy.

You will find you can stay in the position for a long time and it becomes extremely comfortable. Simply breathing in and out through the *Tan Tien* is highly beneficial and meditative.

A 10 MINUTE MIRACLE

Stretches

Here are some simple stretches. Keep within your limits. If you are fit and active, still do them properly and slowly. Do not be tempted to regard them as so basic as not to be worth doing. Each can be used as a 10 minute routine on its own, or you can mix and match them into your own 10 minute warmup miracle.

STRETCH ONE

Stretch your arms above your head, with your palms out, facing upwards. Stretch first to the left, keeping your right foot firm, and stretch along the line of your right leg, hip and body, right up to your hand. Repeat to the left. Then stretch forwards and look up through the gap between your hands (still with palms uppermost). Stand upright again.

Now, interlock the fingers, palms still facing up, and stretch the insides of the wrists alternately. Circle your arms, keeping fingers interlocked – four times clockwise, four times anti-clockwise.

Slowly unlock the fingers, breathing easily and naturally through the *Tan Tien*, and bring your arms down to first position.

STRETCH TWO

From first position, raise arms as before and interlock your fingers above your head. Stretch up as far as you can, even standing on tiptoe if you are able. Then down, then back to first position. Now stretch to the left, keeping your elbows bent and fingers locked, palms uppermost, and keeping your arms above your head. Try to keep your legs as straight and rooted as possible. Bring the arms and head down to the left until they are parallel to the ground. Then come back to an upright position. Now stretch out to the right, pushing your arms straight and looking at your hands. Count to five, then slowly come back up to first position with arms above head. Stretch up, then repeat the side stretch to each side. Do this five times.

STRETCH THREE

Stand with feet together, lean down and place your hands loosely over your knees. Put no pressure or weight on the knee, simply encase your knees with your fingers. Sink down till your thighs are almost parallel to the ground, loosen your shoulders and keep your torso leaning forward. Then make circling movements with the knees, straightening the legs and hamstrings as you go back, bending the knees to the side and front as you go forward. Repeat five times in both directions.

STRETCH FOUR

Stand in first position. Raise your arms, then place your left hand on your right hip, keeping your right arm raised. Breathe normally, then turn to the right following your right hand with your eyes. Twist around as far as you can, then bend, sliding your left hand down along your right leg and keeping your right arm aloft. Stretch as far as you can, then come up, head last. Repeat either side five times.

Focus on the silver string holding you straight as you stand in first posture. Swing your arms, imagining your spine is a central pivot, or a maypole. It remains in the same position, it doesn't bend or sway as you swing your arms and upper torso around, back and forth, as far as you can. Let your arms relax completely and flap around your back if you can. Keep your legs and knees pointing forward.

USING CHI KUNG TO ENHANCE YOUR LIFE

Again, these techniques can be used singly or in tandem with the stretches above or with each other, to create your own 10 minute miracle. Each addresses different aspects of your life – use whichever you feel you need most at any given time.

FIVE 10 MINUTE MIRACLES

Chi Kung for General Strength

Stand in first position and relax. Do not move until you feel you must. Raise your arms and hands, fingers facing each other but not touching, palms facing you. Raise the elbows till they are parallel with the floor and your hands are at chest height. Imagine and feel you are holding a ball of light energy. Feel it resting in your palms. Breathe through the *Tan Tien*. Hold the position for as long as you can.

Chi Kung for the Internal Organs

Stand in first position, breathing through the *Tan Tien*, knees slightly bent. Breathe out and raise your hands to chest height. Straighten your knees and turn your palms outwards as you raise them higher, passing your face. Raise your hands above your head, palms uppermost. Push hands to the sky and stretch your whole body. Come back down in reverse order, breathing in. Finish by breathing out. Do this very slowly 10 times.

Chi Kung for Calm and Stress Relief

This exercise can help calm jangled nerves and develop powerful levels of *Chi* (energy). You can do this anywhere. To begin, move into first position and relax, breathing slowly and deeply but naturally. Do not force your breath. Raise your hands in front of your chest, elbows out, palms facing you. Put your right hand above the left, not touching. Breathe in. Now turn to the left, from the waist, keeping your hips facing forward as much as possible. Twist as far to the left as you can and pause. Now reverse the position of your hands, putting your left hand over the right. Breathe out. Now twist around to the right. Alternate in this way, left and right, for as long as you like. If you wish you can close your eyes or narrow them to slits. This increases the calming effect and helps to centre your energy.

An added option is to meditate or contemplate a situation which is bothering or worrying you. After 10 minutes you will find yourself more peaceful and calm about the situation.

Chi Kung for Confidence and Overcoming Anxiety

This is a form of meditative Chi Kung which focuses *Chi*. Do this first thing in the morning and you will feel the effects long into your day.

Stand in first position. Bring your hands out in front of you and rub the palms together till they are warm. Take your left hand (if you are male) or your right hand (if you are female) and place the centre of your palm on the *Tan Tien*. Now place the palm of your other hand over the first hand so that the centres of the palms are in line with the *Tan Tien*. Stay like this for some time, breathing in through your nose, out through your mouth.

Now gently cup your hands, fingers apart, just in front of the *Tan Tien*, as if you were holding an imaginary ball of light. Let the ball expand and contract, pushing your hands apart or bringing them gently back together. The ball can be enormous and your hands can be wide apart, or it can be the size of a marble, cradled in your cupped (but not touching) hands. Lift your left leg and place it down in front of you. Then and only then allow your weight – and the energy flow – to pass from the right leg to the left. In this manner slowly begin to walk. You can let the *Chi* in your hands pull you or push you in any direction. The ball can grow and diminish. You can bend and twist, holding the ball, feeling the energy grow.

Eventually, let yourself come back to first position. Raise your hands to chest height, palms facing outwards, as if you were stopping something in front of you. Breathe in. Then, breathing out, push your hands further forwards. Feel the *Chi* moving. Bring the arms back and breathe in. Feel the *Chi* attracted to you. Do this slowly five times.

Next, work on the *Chi* to the side of you. Position your hands about one foot in front of your chest, turning the palms first left and then right, pushing the *Chi* gently either side. Do this slowly five times.

Chi Kung for Overall Power

Lie on your back with your feet together and your arms lying by your sides, about a foot from your body. Imagine a golden ball of light travelling down from your head to your toes. As it does so let everything go. Stay this way for a couple of minutes.

Now raise your arms up in front of you as though you were gathering up a large bunch of flowers. Bring the palms right down onto your chest, just below your neck. Place your right hand below your left, both palms pressed onto your chest. Now apply a little pressure and slide both hands down your torso, past the navel. Let the left hand slide under the right. Raise your arms and hands as before and gather flowers. As your hands come down to your chest, place the left hand below your right and then press both palms down along the torso, sliding the right hand under the left at the navel. Repeat.

Do this for five minutes to begin with, or as part of a 10 minute routine such as the one that follows, which incorporates aromatherapy, affirmation, visualization and Chi Kung.

A 10 MINUTE MIRACLE

Combating Problems at Work or School

This routine is designed to help with stressful situations that pertain to your career, working life or life's work at this point in time.

Place 2 drops of Bergamot and 2 of Juniper in a burner. Allow the fragrances to permeate your room or space. Sit in a comfortable position and let yourself relax. Just imagine all the Monday morning turmoil or the prospects of problems you believe you may encounter during the day or have already encountered being purged by the burning oils.

Place a mirror in front of you and focus upon your inner self – through the eyes. Repeat your chosen affirmation three times out loud. Focus all your energy and intention into the affirmation, whatever it may be. Treat it as the most important statement in your life at that moment.

Jot down your reactions. Remember to be honest and

not to edit or alter your very first reaction to the affirmation. This is simple, ongoing 'quality control' if you like. You want to show yourself how your feelings are moving and changing.

Visualization

You are in a great hall. Somehow, intuitively, although you have never seen this place before, you know that outside this room your normal office or factory or school surroundings are just as they always are. You are not alone in the room. At the front, on a great stage, are members of your management team, officials, directors, managers. Now a large crowd is gathering. You recognize many of the faces. You are now in the middle of a great crowd. You are lost in the centre. You become aware that people around you are trying to get themselves noticed. Something important is being decided. You know you have to shine, to stand out, so you do. You let yourself know about all the qualities you have and that you bring to your work. You run through all your successes, however small or trivial they may seem. You remind yourself of all your positive good points. Allow yourself to shine, to feel yourself glowing in the midst of the crowd. When you look down at yourself you see with sudden joy that you are indeed shining like a bright beacon. The light brings an inner confidence you have never felt before.

The crowd begins to melt away before you and you feel yourself being propelled towards the stage. On seeing you everyone starts to smile, then to cheer. You stand before them, your virtue displayed, and you feel safe and warm. Hold the image for a time before letting it fade into your inner storehouse of memories – to be relived at will. You have directed your conscious mind and experienced true visualization. You have not allowed your mind to wander off down daydreaming tracks of wish-fulfilment. Instead, you have filled yourself with positive and health-giving energy.

Chi Kung

Use the 'Confidence and Overcoming Anxiety' (*see page 65*) or the 'Overall Power' (*see page 66*) technique.

When you have finished, shake yourself a little to loosen up. Take a deep breath and open your eyes.

6

CRYSTAL HEALING

ALL ABOUT CRYSTALS

CRYSTALS GAIN THEIR INCREDIBLE ENERGY through long exposure beneath the Earth's surface. Crystals and gemstones can have a very beneficial effect on our lives, transferring some of their energy into our own electro-magnetic field. We actually 'pick up' the healing vibration of crystals and gems.

Some Crystals and Gemstones and Their Healing Properties

Agate	All healing generally, bolsters the ego, attracts good fortune.
Agate (Blue Lace)	Cools, soothes, neutralizes the effects of anger, helps reduce inflammation, fever. Opens throat area.
Green Calcite	Detoxifies the body, good for kidneys, spleen and pancreas.
Amber	Helps earache, bladder, asthma, intestinal, rheumatic problems. Absorbs negative energy, calming. Helps treat depression.
Amethyst	Helps with acne, neuralgia, grief, insomnia. Uplifts and generally heals. Good for meditation too.
Amazonite	Helps meet problems halfway. Helps inner ear imbalances.

Aquamarine	Helps improve sight, nervous system, throat, liver/stomach. Uplifts, calms.
Aventurine	Improves vitality, aids skin disorders. Gives courage.
Beryl	Helps infections of mouth, stomach and throat. Good for liver and heart problems.
Bloodstone	Detoxifies blood and organs, including liver, kidney and spleen. Has a balancing effect on all the chakras (*see page 79*).
Calcite	Helps most ailments.
Calcite (Blue)	Refreshes mentally, spiritually and physically. Relaxes.
Calcite (Gold)	Eases tension away. Lifts depression.
Carnelian	Alleviates rheumatism, arthritis, depression, blood poisoning, nosebleeds. Voice strengthener. Grounding.

Citrine	Helps endocrine and digestive systems, aids circulation, diabetes. Balances emotions, lifts depression.
Diamond	Helps unblock mental anxieties, all negativity.
Emerald	Good memory aid. Has a stabilizing effect. Helps tired eyes. Good for insomniacs.
Fluorite	Grounds, balances, absorbs negative energies and then changes them for the better. Helps all problems relating to teeth; strengthens enamel. Opens chakras.
Garnet	Lifts depression, helps immune system, skin disease. Confidence-booster. Helps imagination to develop.
Kunzite	Balances out negative, emotional, mental anguish. Helps with anaemia, rejuvenates tissue.

Lapis Lazuli	Aids psychic ability and wisdom. Can release old memories. Confidence booster. Good for heart, spleen problems, helps to protect the body from epilepsy and strokes. Cleanses the aura.
Malachite	Helps eyesight, asthma, toothache, rheumatism, erratic periods. Attracts optimism, prosperity. Uplifts, both physically and spiritually.
Moonstone	Helps control of body fluid, water retention. Balances emotions. Aids sensitivity.
Quartz (Clear)	General healer of all ailments. Wonderful air purifier, protective, enhances one's body energy, helps in transmitting energy, storing it, enhancing it and directing it to wherever we wish by simply holding it,

meditating with it and asking for help. Has numerous qualities and nurtures our own intuitive nature. Transmits thought-waves, helps us focus on our goals. Protects us from harmful electrical waves.

Quartz (Rose)   Eases emotional state. Helps you to forgive anyone anything. Aids recovery, uplifts and promotes inner peace and self-worth/love. Helps protect against harmful electrical waves.

Rhodonite   Helps physical energy to return after shock. Helps inner ear, improves hearing. Assists immune system by allowing maximum absorption of vitamins.

Sapphire   Eases nervous conditions. Good for insomniacs. Aids the imagi-nation. Gives peace of mind.

Sodalite	Good for insomniacs. Helps weight control by balancing metabolism. Helps the oversensitive to cope.
Tiger's Eye	Helps ease asthma. Helps creativity of one's own thoughts. Good luck stone, protecting against negative forces.
Topaz (Yellow)	Aids sense of taste. Good for insomniacs. Helps with liver trouble, varicose veins, assists blood vessels. Soothes nerves. A calming stone.
Tourmaline (Green)	Blood pressure regulator. Helps to protect against outside influences of negativity. Aids nervous system.
Tourmaline (Pink)	Helps assist in one's own development, understanding and emotional levels. Balances heart chakra.

| Zircon | Good for insomniacs. All round healing stone. Aids liver. |

The main thing to bear in mind when you buy gems and crystals is that you need to look at them (which appeals most to you?) and touch them (holding the gem or crystal is the best indicator of which one to purchase – you will instinctively feel the one you should have).

Sometimes a gemstone or crystal will catch your eye immediately. Hold the stone and put it down. Then look at a few more – and if you are then drawn back to the stone that first caught your eye, it's probably the one for you.

The Seven Energy Centres

There are areas of the body that take in and give out energy all the time. They are known as chakras in the East. The nearest equivalent in western medicine is the endocrine system. Sometimes these centres are very open and at others they are closed off. The seven chakras of the body are:

1 Base
2 Sacral
3 Solar plexus
4 Heart/thymus
5 Throat
6 Forehead
7 Crown

Figure 1.

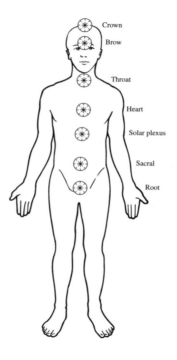

Crown

Brow

Throat

Heart

Solar plexus

Sacral

Root

Here is how the seven main chakras on the body relate to certain gemstones:

1st – Base	Bloodstone, Carnelian, Garnet
2nd – Sacral	Agate, Amber, Citrine
3rd – Solar plexus	Amber (Clear), Citrine, Topaz
4th – { Heart	Tourmaline (Green)
{ Thymus gland	Kunzite, Quartz (Rose)
5th – Throat	Aquamarine, Sapphire, Turquoise
6th – Forehead	Amethyst, Sodalite
7th – Crown	Amethyst, Quartz (Clear)

A 10 MINUTE MIRACLE

Doing a Body Layout with Crystals and Gemstones

Make sure you are completely comfortable, lying down on a bed or on the floor. Playing music softly can sometimes help to create a good atmosphere (*see page 141*). Have the crystals and stones ready in a line.

Over your base chakra place either a carnelian, bloodstone or garnet. Then on the sacral chakra, place the agate, amber, or citrine. Then on the solar plexus place the topaz, citrine or clear amber. And on the heart chakra, some green tourmaline – and so on, until you reach the crown chakra. When your layout is complete, lay very still and meditate. You can do an excellent visualization with the gemstones on your body. Imagine the energy from them penetrating into your field of energy, enhancing and invigorating your whole body.

Stay like this for as long as you feel you want to. And then one by one, take the crystals and gemstones off your body and slowly sit up.

Always remember to wash the crystals and stones in warm water after you use them. You can either dry them with a clean soft towel or allow them to dry naturally, preferably in sunlight.

USING CRYSTALS TO ENHANCE YOUR LIFE

Make sure that you always carry a set of crystals with you, for any occurrence. You can make up a set comprising of a single stone for each chakra (see above). Buy or make a pouch for them, preferably in a dark colour made up of soft material, like velvet, with a drawstring or some other way to prevent them from falling out. Just carrying the crystals with you at all times will allow you to get to know them, and gradually be able to use them as your circumstances require.

Try keeping a set in your drawer at work. When you are feeling low you can place them in a glass dish on top of your desk, between you and the computer for instance, so you can look at them and know that they are helping to protect you. Or use them individually, for instance put the clear quartz crystal in water for a few moments, remove the crystal and then drink the water. You will feel instantly refreshed – your water having been energized.

Wherever you happen to be, **if you feel a bit stressed out**, reach into your travelling gemstone pouch and take out and hold a stone, to help you get back in harmony.

A pick-me-up: Crystals can recharge and energize you. Simply holding a crystal in each hand – pointed end facing outwards from the wrist for the one in your right hand, pointed end facing in towards the wrist for your left. Do this exercise for a few minutes or until you feel completely refreshed. It is a wonderful re-energizer, particularly useful if you are travelling.

For healing muscle and tissue, hold a clear quartz crystal in your right hand and stroke the aura above the injury several times. Try to imagine the aura has little creases or flaws in it and you and your crystal are 'ironing out' these little imperfections. Holding the crystal in your right hand over the thymus gland energizes the body and helps in the repair of muscles and tissue.

For combating low-level radiation, collect several rose quartz crystals and place them around your home or office. Don't forget to collect them up each week, wash them with warm water and a little salt, place them somewhere near sunlight to dry before using them once more. If you like, place them on pink material. They will soak up the wonderful pink energy ray of colour (*see Chapter 8, Colour Healing*).

Adrenalin rush: This happens when we are in a stressful situation, suffering from pressure at work, after an argument, or driving in heavy traffic, especially on a motorway. Adrenalin rush can sometimes occur long after the event. Remove the clear quartz crystal, leaving the other six in their pouch, placing it inside your bra at the front, or in a shirt front pocket. Holding your clear quartz crystal, massage your aura (*see below*), using circular movements, for as long as you are able. Finally, drink a glass of water that has been energized with your crystal. Remove the other gemstones from your pocket.

A 10 MINUTE MIRACLE

The Crystal Massage

Take a clear quartz crystal.

Move it in a clockwise circular motion about six inches away from the body. Imagine the aura as you work the entire length of the body, and the front, back and soles of feet. This is very calming. If you have very little time, say only five minutes, use large flowing circles to get round the whole body. If you have more time, use smaller circles as you move along the aura of the body.

GENERAL SELF-HELP

Tired eyes	Emerald, Malachite, Aquamarine. Take a saucer of water, lay one of these crystals in it for a few minutes and then remove it. Take some cotton wool and gently bathe your eyes with this water. Repeat after a few minutes.
Sore throat	Wear a crystal as a necklace all day. Opaque stones generally tend to absorb their surroundings; semi-opaque are absorbent, but also can transmit

	energy. Match the colour of the stone with those that relate to the throat chakra (*see above*).
When your car breaks down	It is wise always to carry your quartz crystal with you when travelling, especially in your car. The quartz crystal will maximize your car's performance.
Insomnia	Sodalite, Emerald, Yellow Topaz, Sapphire, Zircon.
Asthma	Amber, Tiger's Eye, Malachite. Wear these crystals close to your chest, cleanse them regularly.

A 10 MINUTE MIRACLE

By now you are becoming accustomed to your personal healing space, wherever it may be. You are going to make an affirmation, give yourself a quick crystal massage, then use a combination of crystal power and visualization to create a powerful healing combination. Finally, you can finish off with a couple of Chi Kung stretches.

For this session you will need a clear quartz crystal, an amethyst, an aquamarine, a rose quartz, a clear amber, an agate and a carnelian.

First the affirmation. Place your familiar mirror in front of you and allow yourself to relax. Imagine a golden shower of light descending on and through you. Remember, you may also be practising the affirmation principles and techniques described elsewhere – the 40-day programme, where you are probably homing in on a major key affirmation, repeated every day. You can affirm other aspects of your life during this 10 minute session. One practice will support the other.

In this example, we want to spring clean or purge ourselves of negativity.

You can of course create your own affirmation, but here are some examples:

I am empowered, positive and creative.

I am moving in a positive direction in my life.

I am at one with the crystals. They sweep away all negativity.

Immediately jot down your reaction to the affirmation. Keep these records as a guide to how you are actually feeling.

Arrange your crystals in a line by your side. Nearest you place the clear quartz crystal, then the amethyst, aquamarine, rose quartz, clear amber, agate and finally the carnelian. You will be placing these crystals in this order on the seven body chakras.

Sit in a comfortable position and, taking the clear quartz crystal, give yourself a crystal massage. Hold the crystal and sweep it in circles slowly over your body, as far behind you as you can, keeping the crystal about six inches from your body. You are adjusting and energizing your bodily field, your *Chi*.

When you have finished, lie down comfortably. Place a pillow under your head if it helps, then place the crystals in order as follows:

Base chakra	Carnelian
Sacral chakra	Agate
Solar chakra	Clear Amber
Heart chakra	Rose Quartz
Throat chakra	Aquamarine

Forehead chakra	Amethyst
Crown chakra	Clear Quartz

Relax. Breathe from the solar plexus, gently up to the chest. Imagine the breath circulating around the top of your head and down, in an energy line passing through each crystal.

Visualization

Imagine yourself stepping outside your body, turning around and looking at yourself. Put real power into the thought. Focus on nothing else. When you can hold this image of yourself comfortably, imagine a flow of white healing light entering your left temple. This wonderful energy fills every part of you, pouring into your body like a waterfall. You will notice that, with almost no pressure from you, the white light starts to pour out of the soles of your feet and the stream of healing light follows until your body is part of it. You can focus on any ailment you may have or any condition you may suffer from. As the white light courses through you, let all negative thoughts and emotions go with it.

Carefully remove the crystals from their positions and place them by your side. Don't forget to wash them afterwards and let them dry on a windowsill to recharge.

Chi Kung

Stay where you are and stretch, right down to your toes. Feel your muscles and tendons gently easing out. Now relax and breathe quietly. You can finish off this 10 minute session with Chi Kung Stretch Five (*see page 62*).

7

REFLEXOLOGY

ALL ABOUT REFLEXOLOGY

OUR FEET CAN TELL US WHAT IS HAPPENING throughout our bodies. Reflexology picks up on imbalances in our bodies long before they may be recognized by ourselves or other forms of therapy.

Reflexology works by stimulating the body's self-help mechanisms and the nine body systems (circulatory, digestive, muscular, nervous, respiratory, lymphatic, skeletal, urinary, endocrine). There are over 7,000 nerve endings in the feet alone, and they play a significant part in helping to trigger the body's own healing responses.

There are meridian lines of energy, or *Chi*, running along the entire length of the body. Occasionally there is a hold-up or imbalance, which needs to be unblocked. During reflexology, all the meridian lines that pass through the foot are stimulated and take this message along the route back to your body, helping to create maximum *Chi* energy.

Reflexology promotes a feeling of deep relaxation. Slight discomfort may be felt during treatment, but this is fleeting. A sense of comfort and ease will transport you into a state of calmness. Following a treatment, the body may appear to fluctuate in its response – feelings of sleepiness at first may give way to surges of energy, or a headache may be a way of allowing toxins to leave the body quickly (it is advisable to drink water after, to allow this process). Circulation may be improved. And (like many complementary therapies) reflexology has a balancing effect on these body systems which, after a few hours or days, gives one a sense of well-being.

USING REFLEXOLOGY TO ENHANCE YOUR LIFE

The chart below outlines which areas of the body each region of the feet relates to:

Head and sinuses	Top and sides of all toes
Neck	'Neck' of big toes
Face, mouth, eyes, ears,	Soft pad at the base of the toes
Upper arm	Bony area below the little toe
Upper chest	Ball of the foot
Liver, gall bladder, stomach, kidney (right), adrenal cortex(right), ascending colon,transverse colon	Middle part of the under-foot area (right foot)
Pancreas, stomach, spleen, kidney (left) adrenal cortex(left) transverse colon, descending colon	Middle part of the under-foot area (left foot)

Lower intestine and sciatic belt	Heel of the foot
Knee, hip and shoulder	Outer foot from small toe along to the heel
Spine	Inside area of bottom of foot, from heel to the top of the big toe
Breast, lymphatic and circulation	Top of foot from base of toes to ankles

Figure 2.

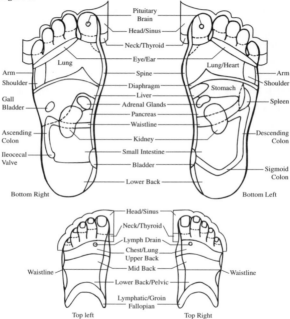

Pituitary
Brain
Head/Sinus
Neck/Thyroid
Eye/Ear
Lung
Lung/Heart
Arm
Shoulder
Arm
Shoulder
Spine
Diaphragm
Liver
Stomach
Gall
Bladder
Adrenal Glands
Pancreas
Spleen
Waistline
Ascending
Colon
Kidney
Descending
Colon
Ileocecal
Valve
Small Intestine
Bladder
Sigmoid
Colon
Lower Back
Bottom Right
Bottom Left

Head/Sinus
Neck/Thyroid
Lymph Drain
Chest/Lung
Upper Back
Waistline
Mid Back
Waistline
Lower Back/Pelvic
Lymphatic/Groin
Fallopian
Top left
Top Right

A 10 MINUTE MIRACLE

A good time to give yourself this workout might be after a shower or bath. Just make yourself comfortable on the floor or on the bed. You might also like to use some foot or body cream afterwards, so it is a good idea to be prepared and have these around you before you begin. Don't forget tissues and a towel to put under your feet so you don't get any oils or cream on the bed or carpet.

Work on one foot at a time. (*Please note:* If you have any heart problems, check with your GP first.) It is usual to start with the right foot, using one or both hands. Sometimes you will have to shift your position slightly to get at the underside or outer edge of your foot. Use rhythmic movements with enough pressure to get the blood supply flowing well, but at the same time go easy on yourself, the pressure doesn't have to be very heavy to get results.

You don't need to spend ages on each area. Try to keep it down to a minimum at first, building up a rhythm to the whole experience rather than concentrating intently on any one area. The idea is to give each foot an enjoyable workout.

With the thumb and forefinger of one hand, take hold of each toe in turn and rotate it several times, first one way, then the other. Gently nip the skin between each toe, first gently and then quite hard, holding the pressure for one second and then releasing. Do this seven times, building up the pressure with each nipping action. At first this area will be a little sensitive, but as you gradually increase the pressure it should ease a bit. Don't feel you have to hurt yourself to gain benefit. Listen to how your body responds. You may have a very sensitive nervous system and therefore the pressure may be just too much, so adjust the pressure accordingly.

Massage the big toe and, using finger pressure, go down each side. Give the big toe a good massage, using a firm pressure all around the front (nail) side and base of the toe. Then massage around the neck of the toe.

Now go along the soft pad at the base of the toes, using firm finger pressure in circular movements. You can use the thumb for this too, or just firm finger-walking. At the outer edge of the foot, under the little toe, using firm pressure, massage on the bony area below the little toe.

For the next movement you need to clench your hand

into a knuckle and work over the ball of your foot, using your knuckles to knead into this area in little movements. You only need do this for a few seconds. If you feel some sore areas, gently work on them until the soreness passes. Don't be too keen to apply lots of pressure.

Now, slide your knuckles down over the high instep area of the underside of your foot, from the ball down to where the heel starts. This whole area (the middle part of the underfoot area) is very sensitive to reflexology – this is because so many of the major organs are represented here.

Go over the whole area of the middle part of the foot, sliding down to the heel and then up to the ball of the foot, being aware of any pain. If there is pain, ease the pressure a little at first and go over that area gently until you feel the pain decrease. Do not do too much to this area, since over-working the reflexes can sometimes over-stimulate the organs and may produce an adverse effect for a short time afterwards – such as feelings of nausea, or a sensation of drowsiness, or too much adrenalin in the system. You may not be able to sleep that night. So please be aware that it is GENTLE pressure you need and you will get good results.

Next, knuckle (or use firmer pressure) and work over the heel on the underside. The area called the sciatic belt runs across the centre of the heel (approximately halfway down). If you have any back problems in the sciatic area, you can help your condition by applying pressure here. Knuckling in a circular action is quite beneficial, but not too hard.

Wring the foot with both hands in a twisting movement (each hand going in a different direction). This action is good for loosening the limbs and spine and is also good for circulation. This should be a fairly brisk but GENTLE action, so that no burning sensation is felt at all, maybe just a slight tingly feeling for a second or two afterwards.

Use a circular motion, with more than one finger if you wish, to massage from the small toe all along to the heel, on the outside of the foot. Keep your fingers in constant contact with one area of skin as you work over it, then lift your fingers and go along a bit further. Continue in this way from the small toe to the heel, and then return along the foot until you reach the small toe again. Repeat once more, going just a little higher on the foot to just below the ankle bone. Remember this is on the outer side of the foot.

Go to the inside of the foot and, using your thumb and a slightly firmer pressure, work along the inside area, noting its curve (similar to the curve of your back). Go up and down this area a couple of times, from the heel to the top of the big toe and back to the heel again.

Now go to the top of your foot and, using all your fingers, massage in small friction movements up and down, evenly and rhythmically (almost as if you were about to scratch the top of your foot – only with your fingertips, not your nails). Don't apply too much pressure here. Work for about 15 seconds. It is a very important part of the workout, so after the friction movement finish off by tracing round the inside and outside ankle bones with your middle fingers a few times. Don't be too firm here.

NOW REPEAT THE ABOVE SEQUENCE ON YOUR OTHER FOOT.

To finish off, start to work in your cream (any good quality foot or hand cream), using upward movements over the upper side of the foot and working around the ankle bones gently as described earlier. Finish off in an upward movement above the ankles towards the knee.

Tips for a Quick Fix

Stiff Neck	Massage around the big toe on both feet and, using thumb and forefinger, circle the toe one way and then the other a few times.
Headache	Work the toes on both feet as described on page 98, not forgetting to massage between each one, paying particular attention to the big toes.
Backache	Work the spine area on both feet, and the heel of the foot, as well as the outer area of the outside of the foot along the heel.

Bad Circulation

An all-over gentle workout is best, paying particular attention to the toes and upper area on both feet. When you have finished, make sure you keep your feet warm.

Hand Reflexology

Your hands have vital reflex points on them, just as your feet do, only they do not appear to be as sensitive to pressure as the feet.

A 10 MINUTE MIRACLE

Hand Reflexology Sequence

This is a great way to boost energy, and can be done almost anywhere.

Shake your hands from the wrists, gently and loosely for a few seconds, to release tension and allow more flexibility.

Start with whichever hand you feel most comfortable. Most of the action of the 'working hand' will be a 'walking finger' movement. Start by taking each finger and gently rotating it a few times, one way then the other, including the thumb. Finger-walk down the sides, top and bottom of each finger in turn (first from the base to the tip and then from the tip to the base). Nip between each finger a few times in the fleshy area between the fingers. Repeat for your other hand.

Next go to the pad at the base of the small finger and, using the thumb of your other hand, press on the area first and rotate on the pressure. Do the same for all the other fingers on this hand, including your thumb.

Go to the outer edge of your palm and, from the wrist, thumb-walk (with the thumb of your other hand) up to the base of the little finger. Go down once more to the wrist, only come in a fraction, and then thumb-walk up to the base of the third finger. Repeat this for the second and first fingers and thumb.

Now, still using the thumb walking technique, go across the palm at the bottom (by the wrist), each time working across at a slightly higher line until you reach the pads at the base of the fingers. Do this last sequence across the palm up to the pads once more.

Turn your hand over and, from the knuckle, gently thumb-walk from the little finger to the wrist. Go back and thumb-walk from the knuckle of the fourth finger to the wrist, then the knuckle of the third finger to the wrist and so on. Repeat this sequence, starting from the knuckle of the little finger once more.

With your working hand, gently encircle and hold your wrist and slowly rotate it, first one way, then the other, several times.

Apply gentle pressure to the outer edge of the knuckle of the little finger and the outer wrist area. Hold the pressure down and make gentle circular movements over the area a few times. Move up slightly and hold the pressure and make circular movements over this area, until you have reached the outer part of the wrist.

With your working thumb, gently press the tip of the little finger, then with your index finger on the nail and your thumb on the back of the top of the little finger, press gently and release, twice. Repeat this sequence along the four fingers and thumb.

Repeat the whole sequence on your other hand.

When you have finished your workout, apply a little hand cream to your hands and relax.

8

COLOUR HEALING

ALL ABOUT COLOUR HEALING

COLOUR IS AN INTRINSIC PART OF OUR LIVES. We absorb the white light of the sun and its healing properties and life-sustaining energy. Human beings are surrounded by an auric field of light. The seven different layers of the aura that surround the human body are like the colours of the rainbow. The quality, depth and vibrancy of this aura very much depends on the physical, mental, emotional and spiritual well-being of the individual.

Colour Survival Guide

★ **Red**   The colour of life, vitality, vibrancy and sexuality; the colour that drives our physical needs. Stimulates, activates the nervous system, encourages adrenalin release in body. Assists blood circulation. Very beneficial for lifting depression. A word of warning: don't overdo the visualization technique (described on pages 120-21) with red – a little goes a long way with this one.

★ **Orange**   The colour of happiness, sunshine and warmth, bringing with it laughter and light to your life. Helps in freeing up mental and physical restrictions; gives courage and the ability to cope with life's problems. Helps cramp or spasms in muscles. Helps to lift the emotions – a very cheerful colour to use. Again a word of warning: just a little at a time. Like the red ray, it is also powerful.

★ **Yellow**   Assists in calming the nervous system and digestive tract. Use this to powerhouse your intellect. A very uplifting colour also. Good for the nervous system and digestive system; and aids in purifying blood. Can assist in helping to balance out one's thoughts.

★ **Green** Works in a balancing and harmonizing way on the body. Just visualizing a green field can help us restore balance to our bodies. It can freshen us up. Great tension reliever, assists when feeling fatigued, in shock, or where there are negative emotions. Has an affinity with the heart – the shade to think of is bright emerald green.

★ **Blue** Cools, slows us down. Can be very beneficial to aid a feeling of calmness and relaxation if one has been over-stimulated in some way. Assists when there is rapid heartbeat, hypertension.

★ **Indigo** Think of this colour as being a deep purple, not as dark as navy blue but with a tinge of red in it to give it that purple hue. Helps cleanse the body of mental fears and allows us to become less inhibited. Cools, purifies blood. Can inhibit bleeding. Helps those with obsessive habits. Should not be used for long periods though, as it can give one the feeling of being anaesthetized. Good for eyes, sense of smell and hearing. Also beneficial on emotional and spiritual levels.

★ **Violet** Assists in helping the nervous system, soothing the entire system. Seems to help on many different levels, mentally, physically and emotionally. Purifies blood. Very calming. Can be a hunger suppressant. Wonderful colour to meditate with.

★ **White** The light of all the seven colours together. If you were to draw on a wheel seven equal segments (as if slicing a circular cake into seven pieces) and coloured each segment with the colours above, then spin the wheel, it would appear white, as the motion of the wheel would allow the seven colours to merge in front of your eyes. Therefore white represents all the colours of the spectrum and is a wonderfully healing vibration that can be used to great effect when visualizing during your self-healing technique.

The seven rainbow colours also correspond to the seven chakras of our bodies (see Chapter 6 for more on chakras):

Red	Base chakra (genital area)
Orange	Sacral chakra (abdominal area)
Yellow	Solar plexus chakra (solar plexus)

Green	Heart chakra (heart/thymus)
Blue	Throat chakra (throat/thyroid)
Indigo	Forehead chakra (pineal gland)
Violet	Crown chakra (pituitary gland)

A 10 MINUTE MIRACLE

Breathing Colour to Heal You

You can sit in a chair if you like, preferably an upright one so you can feel its support on your back. Place your feet on the ground and, closing your eyes, begin to breathe from your diaphragm a few times, each time a little deeper and slower than the last. Do this for a minute or so and then resume a gentle breath. To get the experience of this extremely beneficial meditation with colour, learn to go through the seven colours that correspond with the seven chakras first. You will be amazed at how quickly you will eventually be able to do this and you will be equally amazed at how beneficial it will feel afterwards.

With your eyes closed, see yourself before you, hold this mental picture of yourself and breathing in, take with the breath the colour *Red* directly into your solar plexus and dissipating throughout your body where it is needed.

Next, holding a mental picture of yourself in front of you as before, breathe in and with it take the colour *Orange* into your body. Watch it go into your system, via the abdominal area of your body.

Go through the same process using the *Yellow* ray, watching it flow through your entire body. Again repeat this with the next colour, *Green*. Follow on with *Blue*, then *Indigo* and *Violet*. Finally, concentrate on a *White* light entering the top of your head and cascading down into your body, cleansing your entire system.

When you have got to this stage, sit for a few moments, letting go of your own image once you are satisfied that the colours have been integrated into your whole being. Gently start to focus your attention onto your upright body, sitting in the chair. Become aware of yourself, from your head down to your feet. Once you have done this (a simple 'grounding' technique), it is OK for you to open your eyes. Sit for a moment, take in your surroundings and, in your own time, stand up. Take a glass of water (energized with a crystal preferably – see Chapter 6 on Crystals) and drink it. You should now feel completely refreshed.

By using the colour spectrum in a meditative way like this, we can enhance our etheric layers (outer layers surrounding our body), via the chakras, which then dynamically supercharge our physical body.

USING COLOUR HEALING TO ENHANCE YOUR LIFE

Colour in Everyday Life

Once you begin to meditate with colour, you will instinctively learn which colour you think you need.

Wearing colours can be beneficial to your health. Even choosing a scarf, tie, handkerchief or belt in the colour you need can make a difference to your own well-being.

A good way to keep yourself in tip-top condition is to wear colours next to your skin that will help in the process. (A scarf worn round your midriff, for example).

If you work in a stressful job, or if you have to go some-where and you know you're going to get stressed out, then why not take some colour cards with you? These are small (2-inch/5-cm) square cards you can make yourself. Colour each one with a felt tip pen in one of the rainbow colours. You can do the same thing with a cube or die.

When you are feeling stressed out, take the colour card you think you need – soothing green, calming cooling blue, vibrant red, uplifting yellow, etc. Have the card on your desk and just glance at it whenever you need to. It will not look too obtrusive if anyone sees it and it is just big enough for you to be able to focus on it without drawing too much attention to yourself, or the card.

ENERGIZING YOUR CRYSTALS WITH COLOUR

Simply take a small piece of cloth in the desired colour, or a piece of paper and place it on a windowsill with a clear quartz crystal on top of it. Allow the crystal to take in the energy of the colour (for a minimum of 10 minutes), then use your clear quartz to do a self-massage (*see Chapter 6, Crystal Healing*) or place the crystal in water for a few minutes and then drink the water. You will be doubly charged, not only with crystal energy, but with the healing energy of your chosen colour, taken up and enhanced by the crystal.

EATING THE COLOURS YOU MOST NEED

It may sound funny, but it's true: Colour permeates through the universe and is found everywhere. Colour is a vibration, and the foods we eat, such as plants, berries, fruit, vegetables and meat, all contain it.

Red	fruits or vegetables with red skin, red cabbage, cherries, grapes, radishes, meat, onions, beets
Orange	sweet corn, peaches, tangerines, mandarins, apricots, oranges, pumpkins, carrots
Yellow	sweet corn, yellow skinned vegetables, marrow, carrots,

	apricots, mangoes, grapefruits, egg yolks, butter
Green	fruits and vegetables such as salads, broccoli, Brussels sprouts, cress, leeks
Blue	fish, veal, potatoes, blueberries, plums and other blue fruits
Indigo	as above, also beets, blackberries, aubergines
Violet	as above, and black grapes

Self-help Tips on Colour Healing

On pages 120-21 there's a 10 minute miracle routine for visualizing and meditating with colour. To help you in your choice of which colour to use in this routine, here is a list of problems and the colours which can help to heal them.

| Anaemia | Meditate with the *red* ray for a few minutes. Drink water that has been charged with the red vibration (a colour card |

	underneath a glass of water). Eat as many red fruits and vegetables as you can.
Asthma	Meditate with the *orange* ray for a few minutes, concentrating on the lungs and absorbing the colour there. Using the *blue* ray and imagining it penetrating into the throat area for a few minutes is also helpful. Drink orange-charged water.
Bilious attacks	Charge your drinking water with the *blue* ray and drink at regular intervals.
Bronchitis	Meditating with the *orange* ray and focusing it on the abdomen and stomach areas can be helpful. Drink orange and lemon juice.
Constipation	Concentrate on the stomach and abdomen area for a few minutes as you imagine the

	yellow ray entering your body. Drink yellow-charged water. Do not overdo this treatment, as too much yellow can induce diarrhoea.
Eyes and ears	Meditate with the *indigo* ray and imagine absorbing it into your face and head. Drink water that has been charged with the indigo ray.
Fevers	Where there is inflammation, concentrate the *blue* ray onto this area as you meditate with it.
Insomnia	Meditate with the *violet* ray and take some water that has been energized with that ray to bed with you, drinking some before you attempt to go to sleep.
Nervous disposition	*Yellow* is a very positive ray, and can influence us mentally and physically by being a very stimulating energy. Visualize

	this ray entering the solar plexus. This will not only calm the nerves, but also work on the mental level too, to help get to the root cause of why you feel all wound up.
Promoting a healthy heart	Take in lots of **green** vegetables and fruit. Drink water charged with the green ray. Focus your attention on your heart area when meditating with the green ray and imagine it entering the area.
Sore throat	Concentrate on the **blue** ray as it enters your throat area for a few minutes. Gargling with water that has been charged with the blue ray will help. Do this at regular intervals throughout the day.
Feeling low or sad	Try meditating with the **orange** ray for just a few minutes.
Feeling all fired up	The soothing **green** ray is what

you need to meditate with. It
will help you to balance out your
emotions. Then try using the
blue ray to cool you down and
calm you once more.

When in doubt, just use the pure *white* light to merge
with. Imagine it entering through your solar plexus and
cleansing your entire system of all problems and physical
disharmony.

A 10 MINUTE MIRACLE

Visualizing with Colour

First find a quiet place to sit or lie down. Close your eyes
and start to relax by doing one of the breathing exercises
discussed in the chapters on meditation and visualization.
Allow yourself a few minutes of concentrated, slow, rhyth-

mic breathing and then imagine the colour you wish for self-healing. This can be made a little easier by thinking of a flower in that colour. Gradually you are getting nearer and nearer the bloom until you feel as if you are actually entering into the very centre of the flower. It is so inviting. Focus all the time on its colour ray. Alternatively, think of a large room that has been painted in your chosen colour and imagine everything in that room is exactly the same colour. Wherever you look in the room, all you see is the colour of your choice.

When you can allow yourself more time, a 'combination routine' of affirmation, burning the essential oil(s) of your choice, colour meditation rounded off with a reflexology workout will leave you feeling vibrant and wonderfully healthy.

FINGERTIP HEALING

Pain relief is in your hands.

ALL ABOUT FINGERTIP HEALING

THE SHEER DEXTERITY, COMPLEXITY AND sophistication of the human hand would challenge the skill and ingenuity of the most advanced design engineer. Like your feet, your hands contain patterns of nerve endings and blood vessels beneath the surface of the skin which can be stimulated and triggered into a healing process.

There are other, and cosmically deeper, aspects relating to the design of our hands. Serious palmists will tell you that the distinctive configurations of lines and fingerprints are unique to each individual. Indeed, no two hands are identical. Forensic science has recognized at least one element of this proposition in that we now take fingerprinting for granted; so much so that we forget that it's not just the whorls, loops and other identifying features of our fingertips that are totally unique and the stuff of countless crime novels and TV series. All the other lines, bumps, marks on our hands are also unique to each individual on the planet, even though we share certain basic lines in common – the life line, heart line, head line.

An intriguing belief by many students of clairvoyant palmistry is that the lines on your left hand denote your previous life or incarnation, showing what you bring into your present existence, which in turn is laid out for all to see on your right hand. But you have to know what to look for.

Your hands, and especially your fingertips, can bring you instant pain relief if you know how and where to use them. The therapy required is a blend of shiatsu, acupressure, reflexology and physiotherapy. This may sound complex, but you carry the healing power in your hands. You can teach yourself to heal.

USING FINGERTIP HEALING TO ENHANCE YOUR LIFE

The techniques in this chapter are simple to learn and use. Most of the time you will be concerned with relieving stress of one sort or another – either physical or emotional. You need no special skills, just some basic knowledge. You can get this in 10 minutes, by reading this chapter. Then, use each of the techniques in a 10 minute miracle routine to soothe, recharge and re-energize yourself for life.

SIX 10 MINUTE MIRACLES

For Office Workers

Another busy day. Another stressful day. Very little physical work or exercise, just a slow build-up of stress, toxins, blood pressure rising and nervous anxiety increasing.

To calm yourself, breathe from your solar plexus without inflating your stomach too much. Allow the breathe to push out your ribcage sideways. Keep breathing like this and put your right hand on your chest and your left on your stomach if you're a man (if you're a woman, it's left hand on chest, right on stomach). Try to keep the chest hand flat and let the solar plexus do the breathing, pushing the hand out with the breath.

To relax tension in your shoulders: Place your right hand on your left shoulder, left hand on your right shoulder. Starting at your neck, squeeze the flesh and tendon firmly and hold. Count to three, then move along towards the end of your shoulder inch by inch. Repeat with the other shoulder. Then, using stiff fingers, tap the top of your shoulder and back as far as you can reach comfortably. This stimulates the lymph system and helps clear toxins.

To ease headache: Place the fingertips of both hands behind your neck and, at the base of the cranium, begin small, firm (but gentle) massaging movements. Work your way up the back of your head, spreading out to the temples and back. When you reach the hairline or brow, gently allow your head to be pulled down slightly, stretching your neck.

Computer strain: The real 'Millennium Bug' might be the general strain of working with computers, sitting for hours in front of a flickering screen. Make sure you take adequate breaks. In your breaks, cover your eyes and face with your hands. Breathe out, trapping your breath like a facial sauna, then push your hands up and into your hair. Repeat as often as you wish.

Massage each temple with two fingers. Gently intone a sound or mantra (*see Chapter 4, Meditation*), sub-vocally (to yourself) if you wish. Feel the vibrations of the mantra fluctuate with the rhythm of your massage.

Finally, massage each hand using your thumb, paying particular attention to the wrist. With a twisting movement, place one hand into the other and perform a circular massage on each hand in turn.

Take each finger in turn and gently twist down to the fingertips.

When You Are on the Move

Today we experience a different level of stress and strain to that of our forebears or of people who live a more gentle and tribal way of life. The cause – travel. We all know the situation: driving mile after mile, being stranded on a motorway in a sea of fumes, queuing for a parking space; hanging around the airport, lugging suitcases, children and relatives through crowds so as not to be late; fitting into awkward seats; arriving and going through it all again in a different climate. It's enough to cause any amount of unhealthy stress and toxin build-up. Here are some quick-fix tips.

Nervous headache: Just beneath your skull lies a patchwork quilt of pressure points. Working these points (and there are many key acupressure points running up and down your body) can relieve pressure and therefore pain in key muscle groups and associated bundles of nerve endings. These points are located in a grid pattern. The good news is you don't have to know the precise point before you can massage your scalp. A little bit of experimentation will easily locate the points.

Use your fingertips, spread out slightly and fairly rigid and stiff, to make little circular movements along your forehead, lifting them off the scalp and bringing them down in short, firm jabbing movements. Work your way all over your scalp. This has the effect of stimulating hair growth and reducing pressure build-up which can lead to tense, nervous headaches.

Now pull your hair gently, all over your scalp. Keep the strain on for a count of 10 with each handful. Don't be too hard, but don't be frightened to give it a good tug. Your hair will thank you for it.

Muscular tension in the shoulders: If you have been driving a long way with your shoulders hunched, carrying tension without realizing it, or humping heavy weights such as suitcases, then you could use a way of loosening up.

Find a quiet space (make time for it), inhale into the abdomen and, as you exhale, just let your breath take the weight of your head down to the side. This is not like sports training. It *must* be gentle to avoid overstrain. With the side of your hand, up near your fingertips, make gentle 'chopping' movements along your shoulder from the point below your ear to the edge. This must be a gentle tapping, not a karate chop, or you could do some damage.

Next, rub your hands together to get them warm and tingling, then place them, fingers together, behind your neck. Press and release in a circular movement from the base of your skull to the top of your spine and down either side of the spine as far as you can comfortably reach. Do this four or five times. It's a wonderful rejuvenator. You will find those suitcases feel a lot lighter next time you pick them up.

Stiff jaws, fixed smiles, clenched teeth: Your face tells the story. Look around a typical air terminal, shopping mall or rail station in rush hour (and when isn't it rush hour?). There are the strained faces, the clenched teeth and the tension on display for all to see. Do your face a favour. Find a space. This is always a good start. It means you are taking control and making a commitment. If you are embarrassed, then go somewhere private – the men's/women's room comes to mind.

Begin by patting the underneath of your chin with the backs of your hands.

Then, with your fingertips, tap your face all over, especially around the eyes and temples. Be vigorous and rapid.

Now, pinch the loose skin along your jaw and, starting at the chin, pinch and roll, twist and stretch. You can do this on both sides of the jaw at once. Repeat as many times as you feel necessary.

Blocked ears (in lifts and aeroplanes): Sudden changes in air pressure, such as you might experience in a lift or as an aeroplane takes off or lands, can cause blocked ears. For some people this is a distressing experience.

Sometimes swallowing strongly can help. On most aircraft cabin staff offer boiled sweets to encourage the production of saliva and the urge to swallow. Sometimes people need a little extra help. If you suffer from excessive pressure blockages, try massaging the points just above each jaw bone with two fingers. This is the point just in front of the ears. This has the effect of stimulating the blood vessels and can help release pressure.

Another method is to spread your fingers over your ears, placing the thumb and first two digits behind your ears and the other two in front. If you massage gently in a circular anti-clockwise movement, this will help clear the lymph glands and improve the flow of adrenalin.

Waking Yourself Up

A good way to brighten yourself up is to work on your face. You will probably need to find a quiet corner for this exercise.

Open your mouth as wide as you can and exhale silently in a flow of air. Breathe in through your solar plexus and continue to exhale. Feel the strain on your facial muscles. Now turn this into a silent scream. Let it all out, the tiredness, the irritability and the stress.

Massage in small circles all around your mouth and under your chin. Next, close your mouth tightly and lift your chin, stretching your neck muscles. Repeat these two exercises as you wish. Finally, with partly clenched fists, gently drum all over your scalp. If you can, make the sound *Ahh-Umm* as you do so and let it vibrate around your mouth and then reverberate throughout your body.

If You Can't Sleep

Some shiatsu-style applied finger pressure techniques are exceptionally good at overcoming persistent insomnia.

Press your thumb against the bridge of your nose and hold for about 15 seconds. Lean your head into your thumb in equal pressure to that applied by it. In other words, you are not pressing your head back with your thumb. Let the thumb take the weight of your head.

Another technique is to apply thumb pressure to the hollow just above the wrist, at the side. Hold for 10 or 15 seconds.

You can also grip, hold and slightly massage a point behind your lower leg about 5 inches (12 cm) above your ankle. Squeeze for about 10 seconds. Repeat with other leg.

After a Hard Night

Some of these pressure point applications can ease the worst effects of a night on the tiles or a late meeting followed by a late, heavy meal.

Apart from drinking cold water to combat any dehydration, to relieve headaches, blocked sinuses and lethargy you can use essential oils (*see Chapter 2, Aromatherapy*) to help. Inhale peppermint and use peppermint and lavender to massage the face.

Then you can apply some pressure at two points on the cheekbone. Trace a line with your fingers from the centre of your eyebrow to the points directly under each cheekbone. Press gently and hold. Then massage temples as before.

Press your thumbs against pressure points behind your ears, on the bone of the cranium. Starting with the point nearest the nape of your neck, press each side, edging your thumbs along and up towards the crown until you find the point. It will vary from headache to headache. Now stroke your hands up and down your neck with your head held to one side. Repeat other side.

Backache

Back pain is a widespread ailment afflicting people of nearly all ages and walks of life. A bad back is now virtually endemic and we will all probably suffer one at some time or other. It might be just a twinge, or it might just 'go' and then get better, or it might be something serious. About five million Americans, for example, are partially disabled because of back pain, and another two million can't work as a result of chronic back pain.

Although you can do a great deal to manage, alleviate or cure all kinds of back pain, there are situations in which it will be necessary to take professional advice. Such advice is beyond the scope of this book, but what can be explained are the times when you should consult a specialist:

If your pain is constant and severe and has lasted more than three days of rest.

If it is moderate but has been giving you trouble for more than one month.

If it comes and goes regularly or it affects your bowel movements.

If you get weakness in either or both legs or cannot raise the toes on either foot.

If you lose weight during bouts of back pain or you suffer from any fevers.

If your joints swell or the pain wakes you at night.

Any of these symptoms might mean there is a nerve problem or infection.

You can't beat a bad back by carrying on doing what appears to be causing it. You can't bludgeon your way through it, so if you know what's causing it – stop!

Visualize your pain passing (taking another look at the chapters on Visualization and Reflexology will also help). Find the best position to ease the pain. No two problems are the same, so let your body tell you how to position itself.

Two positions can help. For a spinal disc problem, lie on your stomach, propped up on your elbows to arch the back slightly. If it is a joint problem, then try sitting on the floor with your knees pulled into your chest.

Another good position is to lie on your back and rest your feet and calves on an object such as a chair or the arm of a sofa. Make sure that your thighs are upright, at a 90-degree angle to the floor. Your calves should be horizontal so that you are in a sort of Z-shape. Breathe deeply and calmly.

Stretching

If you can, try stretching by lying flat and allowing your spine to lengthen.

The Arch

Slowly stand up from a sitting position and place your palms in the small of your back, just above the buttocks. Now, lean backwards gently.

Do this a few times till the condition improves.

Push Up

Lie on the floor, on your front with your arms in front of your face. Relax your back muscles using deep breathing. Then get into a push-up position, hands shoulder-width apart. Push up, raising your upper body and leaving your thighs in contact with the floor. Hold for 10 seconds. Repeat as desired.

Knees Up

Lie on your back and raise one leg, bent at the knee. Grasp it with both hands and pull it towards your chest as far as you can, keeping your shoulders and back from raising off the floor. Repeat with your other leg.

Tennis Ball Massage

Lie on the floor with two small (tennis-size) balls under the small of your back on either side of your spine. Breathe deeply and move so that you are rolling along on top of the balls, up and down and from side to side, for as long as you need.

HEALING SOUNDS AND BREATH

ALL ABOUT HEALING SOUNDS

Vibrational Healing with Sound

SOUND IS AND HAS ALWAYS BEEN PART OF A vital communication link: messages sent by drumbeat, Morse code, the pealing of church bells and the acts of praying, singing and chanting all speak to our profound identification with and need for sound.

We rely on so many aspects of sound nowadays. Telephones in offices and businesses, as well as for personal use, have become a way of life – how did we ever live without them? Listening to the radio can be all-absorbing and relaxing – whether it's a play, music or a talk show.

Sounds tell us so much too. If you are on the phone to someone and they are in a public place, you can tell instantly by the level of noise in the background. Noise has become a problem in the late 20th century for some people in their workplace or where they live. Imagine how noisy it must be if you are unfortunate enough to live directly under the flight paths near an airport. Office machinery, sometimes no more than a low-level throbbing noise, can cause distress to some people in their place of work. But even silence can, to some, be an unbearable 'noise'.

To balance all this out, we would do well to be selective about the type of sounds we wish to hear in our free time. We probably already do this to a large extent in the choice of music we listen to at leisure or when travelling to and from work. But we can improve on this quite considerably, enhancing our lives at every given moment, with hardly any extra effort.

There is a vibrational pattern which emanates from sound, occurring everywhere in the environment. These patterns vary in shape (depending on the sound being made), radiate into our own auric field of energy, and cause a reaction to occur. Sound also has a corresponding colour, which acts in much the same way with our bodies.

We can help ourselves in two positive ways with the wonderful vibrations of sound. One way is by listening to sounds that are at harmonic frequencies which enhance our well-being. These harmonic frequencies replicate the very sounds and structure of nature. This 'sound of nature' is called *The Golden Mean*. It was measured and recorded hundreds of years ago by an Italian mathematician called Fibonacci. A sound which correlates to *The Golden Mean* will therefore have a corresponding beneficial and harmonizing effect on a plant, animal, human being – enhancing the existing equilibrium.

The music of J S Bach, for example, has pauses which, when measured, have been found to contain the exact numerical code of *The Golden Mean*. This is wonderful news for all fans of Bach's music, but they probably knew (or sensed) this already. For the rest of us, maybe we should become instantly initiated into the great man's work, for the benefit of our health.

USING VIBRATIONAL HEALING TO ENHANCE YOUR LIFE

The Aim of Sound Vibration

To soothe the energy centres, thereby restoring harmony.

Sound works with colour in the process of helping the body to readjust. Music, known for its ability to raise our spirits when we're down, has healing powers that run even deeper than this.

Symphonic sound is all around us: flowers, trees, shrubs, all emit a keynote – as do we, our planet and the solar system. Funnily enough, the seven-toned musical scale of nature exactly matches that of the seven chakras of the body.

By playing music, we can actually help to develop our chakric centres. As we already know from the earlier chapter on colour healing, the seven centres relate to different colours. When we listen to music that is so pleasing to us, the chakra colours are able to take on a more vibrant intensity. In other words, the symphonic sounds of nature can help to create a clearer colour within each chakra centre.

Base chakra	clear red
2nd (sacral) chakra	deep orange/soft green
3rd (solar plexus) chakra	shimmering gold
4th (heart/thymus) chakra	lemon yellow/cool blue
5th (throat) chakra	azure blue/silver
6th (forehead/'third eye') chakra	yellow/blue/purple
7th (crown) chakra	pure white light

We know instinctively when our nerves are jangled or when we're upset; by playing a favourite piece of music, we can lift and enhance our whole being.

Sounds to Listen To

- ★ J S Bach
- ★ Gregorian chant
- ★ the sea
- ★ early morning birdsong
- ★ the vibrations of a forest
- ★ dolphins
- ★ Indian Ayurvedic vibrational tapes
- ★ whale sounds
- ★ any gentle, peaceful sounds of nature

THREE 10 MINUTE MIRACLES

A Meditation

Select your choice of music, or natural sound. Close your eyes and get comfortable in a chair or on the floor or bed, making sure you won't be disturbed.

*Allow the sounds of your choice to waft over and around you
for a little while. Now imagine that you are the music, you
are the sea, forest, dolphin or whale. Just be ... allow yourself
to be that part of nature ... Release your own boundaries
and experience.*

*When the tape finishes or you feel you have had enough,
withdraw back into your own body, becoming aware of your
limbs, torso, head, neck, feet, hands, fingers and toes. Gradually
open your eyes when you feel ready, and slowly stretch.*

Waterfall

Try this meditation to the sound of a waterfall and the natural vibrations of the forest.

This is a very cleansing therapy. Settle yourself as
before.

*Imagine you are waist-deep in a beautiful lake deep in a
forest, completely alone. There is a waterfall close by and you
swim over to it. The water is wonderfully cool on this hot
day. Standing under the waterfall, you feel the gentle shower
of water as it cascades down over your head, shoulders and*

body, like pure silver raindrops. Stay there as long as you feel
you need to. When you feel you have had enough, imagine
you are out of the water now, dry from the warmth of the
sun. Gradually become aware of the room you are in. When
ready, open your eyes and slowly stretch.

Visualization

Select your choice of calming music. Close your eyes and
settle down as before and begin to allow yourself to float as
you listen to the music.

When you feel ready, imagine each time you breathe in that
you are absorbing the pure vibration and colour from
the music. The deeper notes denote RED and ORANGE. The
middle notes denote YELLOW, GREEN and BLUE and
the higher notes, TURQUOISE, MAGENTA and PURPLE.
The very top notes relate to WHITE.

So each time the deeper notes are played, imagine them
entering your base and second chakra with red and orange
colour. Then, when you hear the middle notes of the music,

imagine the yellow, green and blue rays to enter your solar plexus, heart and throat chakras. When the higher notes are played, allow the turquoise, magenta and purple rays to enter your third eye or sixth chakra. And when the very top notes are played, imagine the pure white vibration of light entering your crown chakra.

This is not an easy technique and is one you may well have to build up to (it is helpful if you are already quite familiar with the music or sounds you are going to work with), but is very rewarding once you have mastered the technique.

Sounds Amazing

The second way we can use sound to maximize health is to use our voices to create harmonic vibration.

To chant continuously, voicing a word or words repeatedly over a given period, creates harmony within the body. The resonance of the chant gradually induces a change, not only in the structure of the mouth itself, but also in the torso and eventually in the whole body, resulting in a change of activity at cellular level, thereby harmonizing the body's systems and creating a pure vibration of rhythm. And that's a scientific fact!

Chanting can relate to the base chakra initially, gradually elevating through to the higher levels and the crown chakra.

FIVE 10 MINUTE MIRACLES

House Clearance

Houses that have not been lived in for a while seem to decay quickly, not simply through lack of maintenance, but more a lack of interactivity and the vibration of love from its owners.

To rid a house of unwanted or heavy vibrations, or if a house hasn't been lived in for a while and it feels a bit creepy, here's what to do.

Put on a favourite piece of music.

Go round each room, open the windows and clap your

hands, chant, and sing. Hold a clear quartz crystal and imagine a gossamer-light net attached to it. Walk round the room making slow sweeping movements in the air 'trawling' up the negative energy. Cleanse the crystal immediately after use.

To Calm Down

Interconnect your mind, body and spirit if you feel at a low ebb, or have been doing too much cerebral thinking and can't sleep.

Chant – any rhythmic repetitive word or words, at your own pace. *OHMMM* is a good one to start with.

Hum – one note can resonate in your upper body and produce a feeling of calmness. This is particularly calming following an argument or altercation.

Combating Loneliness or Fear

Take any opportunity to sing. This can be along with the voices on a tape or the radio or TV. This is helpful if you feel a bit lonely or detached from life, due to stress, or if you work from home or live alone. It helps you to feel connected with yourself and also with others, who for whatever reason are not with you in your hour of need.

Singing actually assists in connecting you to your own emotions once more.

Whistling

Whistle a happy tune – just as Anna advised her son in *The King and I*. It 'breaks' the spell of an atmosphere when you are confronted by anyone or anything you are unsure of.

Interviews and Important Meetings

Having a good clear voice can be a very important plus if you're going for an interview. Tone of voice is very important. How you voice your answers to a question could be a deciding factor in whether you are successful or not. Voices can sound intimidating, commanding, powerful, weak, soft, silly, depressing, uplifting, funny or humorous to the listener. Before an interview, listen to your own voice (on tape) at home and keep re-recording the same words until you feel satisfied. Remember, different sounds create different shapes and colour – you want to create the very best shape and colour for your own life and those around you, for maximum chances in the workplace, with your family and friends, and in all key areas in your life.